Integrating Therapeutic Play Into Nursing and Allied Health Practice

Judi A. Parson • Belinda J. Dean
Natalie A. Hadiprodjo
Editors

Integrating Therapeutic Play Into Nursing and Allied Health Practice

A Developmentally Sensitive Approach to Communicating with Children

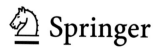 Springer

Editors
Judi A. Parson 🆔
School of Health and Social Development
Deakin University
Geelong, VIC, Australia

Belinda J. Dean
School of Health and Social Development
Deakin University
Geelong, VIC, Australia

Natalie A. Hadiprodjo
School of Health and Social Development
Deakin University
Geelong, VIC, Australia

ISBN 978-3-031-16937-3   ISBN 978-3-031-16938-0   (eBook)
https://doi.org/10.1007/978-3-031-16938-0

This Springer imprint is published by the registered company Springer Nature Switzerland AG
The registered company address is: Gewerbestrasse 11, 6330 Cham, Switzerland

We would like to honour and celebrate our families.

Judi would like to celebrate appreciation for her partner, John, and son, Izaak, thank you for being so patient with me as I pursue my passion for all things play.

To my parents for providing me the ultimate childhood and giving me a solid foundation to raise my own kids. To my kids for all the joy and challenges! You've taught me more than I could have ever imagined! Belinda Natalie would like to share her gratitude for her parents, siblings, and a play-filled childhood and appreciation for her husband Nugi. Thank you for your love and support.

Foreword

Healthcare professionals, nurses, and allied health practitioners are heroic individuals who are often called upon to deal with all manner of medical situations. They are often on the frontlines and become severely impacted by the trauma situations they encounter. Their skills and endurance have been tested and taxed in the recent past in dealing non-stop with a myriad of health issues that have erupted from a pandemic that has impacted the world and people of all ages. They are required to offer sensitive and difficult care ranging from assessing the sick to supporting a dying child.

Those nurses and allied healthcare professionals need even greater sensitivity when working in paediatric care. These patients' developmental levels require thinking out of the box and bringing in playful and play-based means of helping to deal with pain, difficult and frightening procedures, separation, and dying. Those who work in paediatrics are required to have expertise at a unique level of understanding, support, and generalized developmentally sensitive knowledge of child development, neuroscience, and attachment, along with the health model. Often self-care is overlooked and time for specialized and supportive training is lacking.

On the other side are the parents who are dealing with their child's health issues and seeking medical professionals who are knowledgeable and sensitive. As a parent you wish the best for your children: good health, happiness, love, and prosperity. But life is often a roller coaster ride with unexpected turns and dips. It has a way of throwing us a curve ball and when it comes to our children's health sometimes the outcome can be traumatic for the child, for the parent, or for both. Even when children visit a doctor for wellness checkups, they may become anxious and stressed by the visit. Many aspects of the visit with the doctor can be threatening or uncomfortable, from being held by unfamiliar people and having their movement restricted to receiving shots. Such routine visits can have long-term effects of anxiety and stress on the child. Depending on the developmental stage, the child is in their understanding and reaction to the everyday experience of a doctor's visit may become confusing and difficult to understand.

When a child has to be hospitalized, have surgery, or has a chronic congenital medical problem, the stress and anxiety associated with their treatment and separation from their parent, home, school, and familiar surroundings is magnified exponentially. The long-term impact is substantial, not only on the child but on the parent as well. The child and even teen can have difficulty understanding the complex medical procedures and events that are occurring or they will be experiencing. Their ability to communicate their pain and hurt can be significantly limited, and their conceptualization of why things are happening to them may become distorted and confused.

It has long been recognized that play is the work of children and the means through which they process difficult experiences. Allowing a child to play is one of the most powerful and effective means of reducing children's stress and increasing empowerment. Play is a means through which children act out and process unpleasant experiences and minimize resulting negative psychological impact. We know from research and the abundance of available writings that play has therapeutic and healing properties. We can gain valuable insight into children's emotional states through their play. When a child feels safe enough to express and play out a variety of feelings, the negative feelings brought on by past and current unpleasant medical experiences can be processed. Most children need very little encouragement to participate in dramatic medical play and make use of play-based activities. Children are readily drawn into play situations, with play as their most natural and major means of communication. Nurses and allied health practitioners can help and encourage children and teens with medical issues to talk, play, and process their feelings and concerns, along with helping them to sort out their perceptions, understanding, and knowledge of what is going on. Medical dramatic play allows a window into the child's feelings and can help reinforce correct information about medical care.

The therapeutic powers of play through planned medical play activities and therapeutic play can allow children to participate actively in a learning process that helps them to better understand what has happened to them or to become familiar with impending procedures. Dramatic medical play allows children the chance to handle various medical equipment, and it provides opportunities for rehearsing, becoming desensitized to, and expressing feelings related to the medical experience. It can become an empowering experience that can build self-esteem and self-expression.

No one wants to see a child in pain or upset or feeling helpless in the face of medical procedures. We want to be able to offer support and emotional comfort. We want to have the tools necessary to use in our therapeutic work. *Integrating Therapeutic Play into Nursing and Allied Health Practice: A Developmentally Sensitive Approach to Communicating with Children* is that timely tool, with knowledge and resources, offering the best of both worlds: ways to increase paediatric knowledge as well as how to sensitively address the needs of parents and children. Readers learn new ways to engage young patients through therapeutic play, being attuned to the parents' needs, as well as considering the importance of professionals addressing their own need for self-care. This unique volume offers practical information along with the weaving in of dynamic interventions to address the child and adolescent's physical, psychosocial, neurological, and cognitive development with therapeutic play and play-based considerations. The authors have also offered poignant case studies that get to the heart of what it is like for the child to deal with issues of short-term acute events, chronic pain, abuse and neglect, chronic medical diseases, mental health issues, and impending death. These case studies give us a unique perspective into the world of the child and how best to address them on a practical level with greater sensitivity along with ways to significantly optimize paediatric care.

How glad I am that such a volume is available today for nurses, allied health professionals, and other professionals on the care team. This unique volume will assist them in helping the myriad of children and teens coping with health issues benefit from the therapeutic activities! You will find this book becoming a much-used tool in your professional toolbox!

Athena A. Drewes
Formerly Clinical Director of Training and Director
of the American Psychological Association
Doctoral Psychology Internship at Astor Services for
Children and Families in New York

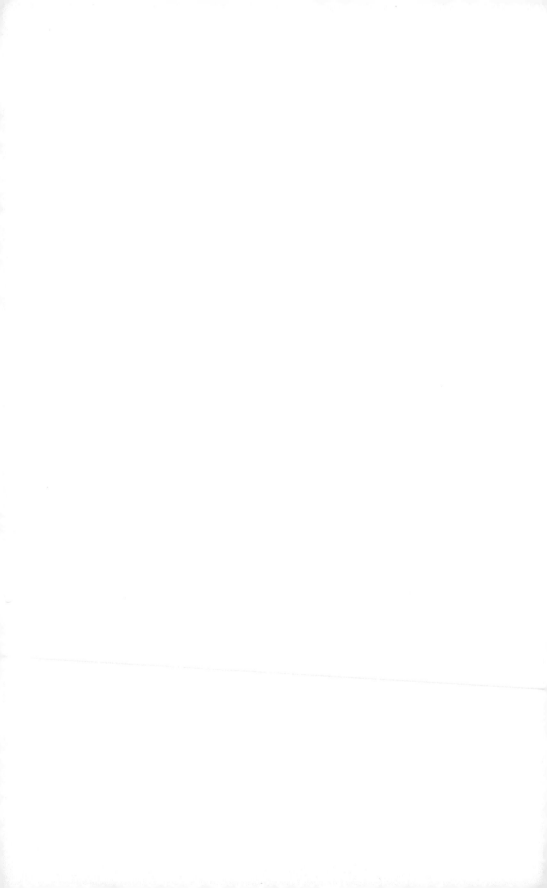

Preface

This text aims to support developmentally sensitive nursing and allied health care by integrating the therapeutic powers of play into child and adolescent health service provision. It is designed to link play, child development, neuroscience, biopsychosocial, and attachment theories with the biomedical model of health.

Nurses and allied health practitioners care for children aged between 0 and 18 years and with diverse childhood illnesses, injuries, diseases, disorders, and conditions, and are therefore in a prime position to understand and support children and adolescents through potentially painful and traumatic healthcare experiences. Understanding of the role of play and the application of the therapeutic powers of play in communicating with children and families has the potential to significantly optimize paediatric care.

The theory that supports play-based strategies, tools, and techniques presented in this text will assist nurses and other health professionals to engage with children in an age-appropriate manner and 'speak' with children through their natural language of play to enhance comprehension coping, resiliency, and healing. Play is recognized as a sequentially developing ability and can be aligned with the child's age and stage of life. Play-based approaches can be placed on a continuum from fully child led or non-directive play to adult facilitated educative play. Medical information can be tailored according to the various points along this continuum to inform clinical reasoning and to help children prepare for procedures, recover from medical interventions, and/or make sense of their diagnosis.

Whilst the book is primarily directed at nurses and allied healthcare professionals who work with children and their families, it may also be a valuable resource for medical and other kindred professionals, who work together as a team. The reader will be introduced to various strategies to illustrate how to playfully engage children through a range of case vignettes.

Enjoy reading.

Geelong, VIC, Australia   Judi A. Parson
Geelong, VIC, Australia   Belinda J. Dean
Geelong, VIC, Australia   Natalie A. Hadiprodjo

Contents

Editors and Contributors

About the Editors

Judi A. Parson PhD, is a paediatric qualified Registered Nurse, Play Therapist/ Supervisor, and Senior Lecturer/Discipline leader for Play Therapy, School of Health and Social Development at Deakin University, Australia. Her doctoral thesis focused on the integration of procedural play for children undergoing invasive medical treatment. She completed her Master of Play Therapy (with Distinction), through Roehampton University London, and is actively involved in the development of play therapy in Australia. Judi, a co-founding director of the Australasia Pacific Play Therapy Association (APPTA) and a founding member of the International Consortium of Play Therapy Associations (IC-PTA), continues to practice play therapy and provide clinical and research supervision to others in the field of paediatrics and play therapy. She has published more than 40 book chapters and journal publications and co-edited Prendiville & Parson (2021) *Clinical applications of the therapeutic powers of play: Case studies in child and adolescent psychotherapy* Routledge.

Belinda J. Dean (BA, MA, RND1, RPT) is a qualified Registered Nurse, Registered Play Therapist, Lecturer in Child Play Therapy, and PhD candidate at Deakin University. Belinda has 22 years of experience in the healthcare field with a focus on Child and Adolescent Health and Development, Mental Health, Community, and Family Health. Belinda lecturers in the above areas including educating students around Medical and Procedural play. Belinda holds a Master of Child Play Therapy and supervises postgraduate Play Therapy students and alumni. Belinda is passionate about play-based modalities to support individuals, families, and wider systems. Belinda practices integrative play therapy with an attachment and trauma lens, incorporating Medical Play Therapy approaches, Learn to Play Therapy, Child Centred Play Therapy, and Filial Therapy modalities. Belinda is a past facilitator of the Imagine, Create, Belong program and has co-authored *Storying Beyond Social Difficulties with Neuro-Diverse Adolescents* manual and related published peer-reviewed papers and presents and provides training nationally on this research. Other areas of research include integrating therapeutic play-based approaches into higher education, nursing, and allied health care. Belinda continually ensures that she is holding the child in mind non-judgementally and with a continual unconditional positive regard. Belinda extends this to keep in mind unconditionally the child's background, culture, family situation, and development. Belinda is the director of Light Heart Play Therapy and a practicing play therapist.

Natalie A. Hadiprodjo PhD, is a registered Play Therapist and Supervisor. She is the Course Director for the Therapeutic Child Play and Master of Child Play Therapy postgraduate programs within the School of Health and Social Development at Deakin University, Australia. Natalie completed a Bachelor of Occupational Therapy at the University of Queensland, a Master of Counselling at the Queensland University of Technology, and a Master of Play Therapy (with Distinction) and PhD, through the University of Roehampton, London. She was awarded the Psychology Department Prize for Outstanding Achievement for her master's thesis and built on this work in her doctoral research integrating the fields of attachment, trauma, and play therapy. Her doctoral research explored the novel application of physiological monitoring to play therapy research. Natalie has presented this research internationally in the UK, Europe, and Australia. Natalie has 20 years of clinical experience and has worked across mental health, paediatric, and educational settings in Australia and London. She is actively involved in the development of play therapy in Australia through education, research, and clinical and research supervision within the field of play therapy.

About the Contributors

Rhiannon Breguet is a qualified and registered Play Therapist/Private Practitioner/ Causal Academic within the Master of Child Play Therapy program, School of Health and Social Development at Deakin University Australia and Play Therapy Clinical Supervisor and member of the Australasia Pacific Play Therapy Association (APPTA). She completed her Master of Child Play Therapy at Deakin University Australia. Prior to her qualifications in Child Play Therapy, Rhiannon enjoyed 12 years working with children, families, and carers in the Out of Home Care sector. Rhiannon co-presented a paper, titled *Creating a Therapeutic Experience for Children in Out of Home Care during Contact with Birth Families* at the World Health Association for Childhood and Infant Mental Health conference in Cape Town, South Africa. Rhiannon previously worked in the Catholic education system as a Play Therapist. Rhiannon's particular area of interest is trauma and working with vulnerable children within the child protection system.

Erin Butler has completed a Bachelor of Education (Early Childhood) and an MA in Play Therapy (with Distinction). Erin has extensive experience in Australia and the UK educating and providing therapeutic support to a diverse range of children. She began her career as an Early Childhood/ Primary School Teacher (birth to 12 years of age), working in a variety of educational settings. Erin has since gained a wide range of clinical experience as a Play Therapist (3–15 years of age) and Child

Life Therapist (birth to 19 years of age), primarily working in schools and community healthcare settings, such as a bereavement and loss service, Play Therapy charity, and children's hospice.Erin researched the role of Child-Centred Play Therapy for children with a chronic or life-limiting illness whilst studying at the University of Roehampton, London. This research explored the importance of the therapeutic relationship when working within a range of family contexts and community settings. She presented her findings at the 2019 APPTA Conference in Brisbane, Australia.Erin is committed to the growth of Play Therapy in Australia and has also been employed as a Casual Academic and Clinical Supervisor for the *Master of Child Play Therapy* program at Deakin University.

Athena A. Drewes PsyD, MA, RPT-S, is a licensed psychologist, certified school psychologist, and Registered Play Therapist and Supervisor. Formerly Clinical Director of Training and Director of the American Psychological Association Doctoral Psychology Internship at Astor Services for Children and Families in New York. She currently lives in Ocala, FL. She has over 45 years of clinical and supervision experience with complex trauma, sexual abuse, foster care children and adolescents, in school, outpatient and inpatient settings. She is former Board of Director of the Association for Play Therapy and Founder and President Emeritus of the NY Association for Play Therapy. She is a frequently invited guest lecturer around the United States and internationally around the world, including Canada, England, Ireland, Italy, Argentina, Mexico, Australia, Taiwan, Denmark, Korea, and China. She has published numerous book chapters, journal articles, and edited/co-edited 13 play therapy books with the most recent play-based interventions for childhood anxieties, fears, and phobias; puppet play therapy; play therapy in middle childhood with a companion DVD of Dr Drewes demonstrating her work in Prescriptive Integrative Play Therapy with the American Psychological Association; and co-edited with Dr Charles Schaefer *The Therapeutic Powers of Play: 20 Core Agents of Change*.

Dolores Dooley MHlthSc (Edu), BN(Hons), RN, RM, Dolores Dooley is a lecturer in the School of Nursing and Midwifery at Deakin University Victoria. She has extensive clinical experience in midwifery, paediatrics, and neonatal nursing. Dolores has published in the area of nursing and midwifery students understanding of emotional intelligence. Her teaching interests include supporting student nurses and midwives, so they have the knowledge and skills to work with parents to enhance infant well-being and strengthen parent–infant relationships.

Phoebe Godfrey holds her master's degrees and is qualified and registered as both an Occupational Therapist (with AHPRA) and Play Therapist (with APPTA). She works currently as a private practitioner and founder of Together in Play, as well as a Lecturer in Child Play Therapy at Deakin University. Prior to this working as a casual academic following her master's completion, in both marking and supervising postgraduate Child Play Therapy students at Deakin University. In addition, Phoebe has 10 years of experience in working as an aquatic educator, with a key focus in supporting children living with additional needs in their connection to self and the joy and safety within an aquatic environment. Her hard work and dedication in this area was recognized when she received both the AUSTSWIM Victorian and National Teacher of Access and Inclusion awards in 2019. Phoebe continues to stay in this space which seamlessly compliments her work in clinical practice and within her teaching and support roles with Deakin university. Her interest lies in the heart of emotional development. Clinically, her work aims to build and maintain positive relationships and connection to self, others, and environment to be able to empower children and families to have fulfilling and positive relationships and experiences, increase functional capacity and joy in their individual journeys, and ultimately reach their full potential. Likewise, with students her focus is on increasing and supporting them to create meaningful connections within their studies and to confidently walk their own path of learning and passions within the field of Child Play Therapy.

Leanne Hallowell MEd (Melb) is a Lecturer in the Faculty of Education and Arts at Australian Catholic University (ACU) and is a PhD candidate at the University of Melbourne. Leanne was originally qualified as an early childhood teacher before moving into what was then known as Educational Play Therapy at the Royal Children's Hospital (RCH) in Melbourne, Australia, as the Head of the Department.

Leanne's worked at RCH in various emergency departments: with children with a diagnosis of cystic fibrosis, with children requiring liver transplantation, and in radiology. Work in radiology included the development of a program to support children to undergo an MRI without the use of anaesthetic. The team working on this project won state government awards for excellence in paediatric health care and internationally for clinical practice in radiology.

Leanne's current research describes and theorizes effective engagement and interventions with children in medical settings in particular in relation to understandings of medical interventions and procedures. Most recently, this work has focused on capacity-building amongst medical and allied health professionals in healthcare settings in ways to support children's understandings of impending medical procedures and ways in which children may be supported to be active participants in their own health care. In particular, with a focus on how communication is best managed in paediatric settings. Leanne has also worked as a consultant with architectural firms on supportive environments in paediatric health care and educational settings.

Sarah Hickson holds a Bachelor of Social Science and Master of Arts Play Therapy (with distinction). She works in private practice as a Play Therapist in London, UK. Sarah has over 25 years of experience working with children from various backgrounds and is specialized working with children and families who have experienced significant trauma and attachment disruptions, with a particular interest working with adopted children. Sarah also supervises other Play Therapists from across the globe and is a director on the board of The British Association of Play Therapists.

Fiona M. Melita MCPT, APPTA- RPT, RN (Non-Practicing) is a Registered Play Therapist. She is the founder and director of *Becoming Me Play Therapy (BMPT)*, a private practice in Townsville, Queensland, offering play therapy services to children and families. She holds a Master of Child Play Therapy from Deakin University, a Bachelor of Health—Nursing (with Distinction) from Central Queensland University and has practiced as a Registered Nurse for Queensland Health in General Medical, General Surgical, Oncology, and other areas. She also holds an Associate Diploma of Education (Child Care) and has worked in the childcare industry in Australia and primary schools in London, UK.

Michelle Perrin BEd; Grad. Dip Health Management; Certified Infant Massage Instructor. Michelle is a Child Life Therapist working in a tertiary Children's Hospital in Newcastle, Australia. She has 21 years of experience working with children with acute and chronic healthcare needs. Michelle is currently doing her Master of Play Therapy to further enhance her skills in this area. She has also worked as an educator for young children with Autism.

Michelle has a strong interest in paediatric procedural care support. She is passionate about empowering children and their families to manage their hospital experience and reduce their perception of pain. She has previously held the position of Chair of the Association of Child Life Therapists Australia (ACLTA) and is actively involved in supporting the growth of the Child Life profession in Australia.

Kerry Reid-Searl AM (PhD, RN, RM, MClin Ed, MRCNA, FCN) is an Emeritus Professor at CQUniversity, a Professor of Innovation and Simulation at the University of Tasmania and an Adjunct Professor at Monash University. She has been a paediatric nurse for over 20 years. Kerry has been involved in undergraduate nursing education at CQUniversity for 32 years. She has extensive teaching experience and has developed two simulation techniques termed Mask Ed and Pup Ed. These innovative teaching techniques focus on patient-centred care and allow learners to experience humanistic and realistic simulation experiences in the most innovative way. The techniques are now used across the world. Kerry has been the recipient of numerous teaching awards. Some of these include the CQUniversity Vice Chancellors Teaching Award in 2008 and 2010, a Faculty of Science Engineering and Health teaching award in 2008 and 2010, an Australian Learning and Teaching Citation for her outstanding contribution to student learning in 2008 and 2012, was named Pearson/Australian Nurse Teacher Society—Nurse Teacher of the Year in 2009 and in 2012 was awarded and Australian University Teaching Excellence Award. In 2013, Kerry received the Simulation Australia Achievement Award. She has received four CQUniversity Opal awards for innovation and research. In 2019, she was awarded a member of the order of Australia for her contribution to nursing education. Kerry is well published in international journals for her work. She has delivered an extensive number of keynote and/or invited speaker presentations globally and has been the principal author as well as co-author of several nursing textbooks.

Kate L. Renshaw B Psych, Grad. Cert. HELT, Grad. Dip. Art Therapy, Grad. Dip. Play Therapy and PhD Candidate. Kate is a Play and Filial Therapist and academic at Deakin University. She holds registrations with BAPT (Registered Play Therapist), APPTA (RPT/S), and APT (International Professional). Kate works therapeutically with children, families, and teachers and offers Play Therapy Clinical Supervision.

Bridget Sarah MCPT, BOccThy (Hons), Grad. Cert. HELT, APPTA RPT. Bridget is a Lecturer and Researcher in the Master of Child Play Therapy, School of Health and Social Development at Deakin University, Australia. She is an Occupational Therapist and Play Therapist who has worked with children with a range of physical and cognitive developmental disorders and delays in each home, school, and community-based settings. Bridget is passionate about the provision of developmentally sensitive and psychotherapeutic interventions for children and their families with complex care needs.

Karen Stagnitti is Emeritus Professor in the School of Health and Social Development at Deakin University, Geelong Australia. She has researched play, play assessment, and how to build children's pretend play ability since the early 1990s. She has over 140 publications.

Part I
Theoretical Background

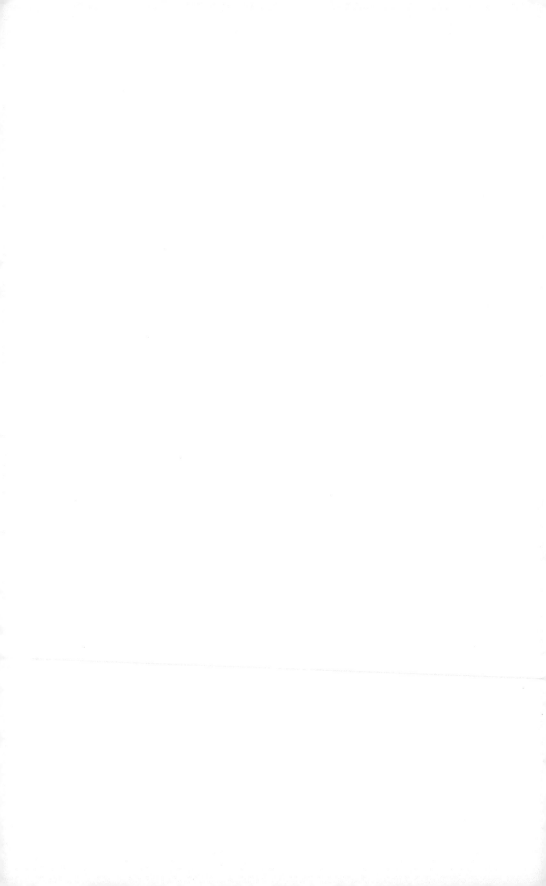

Integrating Play into the Context of Health Settings

Judi A. Parson, Fiona M. Melita, and Belinda J. Dean

Objectives

At the end of this chapter, you will be able to:

- Discuss the importance of play.
- Differentiate play and play therapy.
- Explain the benefits of play as a therapeutic tool.
- Reflect on the rights of the child in the context of health settings.

Introduction

Integrating therapeutic play into nursing and allied health care may at first seem incongruent. However, this text positions the healing powers of play as the central feature to not only strengthen communication with children in a developmentally sensitive way but to prioritise play as a human right. Incorporating a humanistic stance, the professional positions their work with children and adolescents in a developmentally sensitive and client centred way. To do this the professional is cognisant of the age and stage of development, the critical factors that may impact on the child in relation to the child's lived experience in relation to their concerns and within the health setting.

J. A. Parson (✉) · B. J. Dean
School of Health and Social Development, Deakin University, Geelong, VIC, Australia
e-mail: judi.parson@deakin.edu.au

F. M. Melita
Becoming Me Play Therapy (BMPT), Townsville, QLD, Australia

The authors of this chapter are all nurses who have worked with children, adolescents and families in a variety of health care settings. They also hold master level qualifications in Play Therapy. This knowledge provides pivotal insights at the intersections between paediatric nursing, mental health, play, and play therapy. Parson [1] through doctoral studies explored the factors that facilitated or inhibited nurses use of procedural play when children with cystic fibrosis underwent medical procedures. In this study, most nurses had an implicit understanding of play, but not an explicit discourse of play [1]. Another key finding was that procedural play was a silenced discourse in paediatric nursing. Procedural play is mix of developmentally sensitive, educative and therapeutic play. Play is understood as the child's way of communicating what he or she knows about the world and therefore it makes sense to integrate play into nursing and allied health care as a specific adjunct to facilitate communication.

The Importance of Play

There is no consensus on the definition or importance of play. Play to one, may be work to another, invaluable to some, and frivolous to others. Regardless of opinion, research and observation has given reason and purpose to play, and negative outcomes are acknowledged when play is limited or absent in the life of both animals and people [2]. The associated problems with a lack of play highlight that play must possess powers. Brian Sutton-Smith [3] proposes that each discipline seeks and finds purpose in play through the lens of their interest. Perhaps then, rather than offer another disciplines perspective of play, we should seek to understand what it means to the individual. The many lenses and purposes offered already suggest that play is unique to each. Where else than in the field of play therapy where we seek to understand the client's world through their eyes [4] could an individual perspective be more suited. Can we decide that another person is not playing because we cannot find the joy in what they do? And perhaps that is where we make the distinction. Everyone is different. What is play to the individual? After all, recognising this is what will interest and motivate a client, help to identify appropriate forms of distraction and relaxation for them, and bring those moments of positive emotions that support therapeutic change. So, what is play to you, and what is it for the client?

The important thing is not what we play, it is that we play, and more importantly with others. In the animal world, distinct deficits in social skills and emotional intelligence are found in 'social mammals' when play opportunities have been restricted [2]. Studies with rats have shown that isolation and deprivation of rough and tumble play in the early years resulted in abnormal social and sexual behaviour, and aggression in later years [5]. Brown [6] discusses interviews with thousands of individuals that found maladaptive coping, self-regulation difficulties, aggression, and interpersonal relationship issues in later life were associated with ongoing moderate to severe play deprivation in the first 10 years of life. He also identifies play deprivation as a common theme, amongst others, in the histories of many mass murderers [6] and homicidal males [7]. The value of play is apparent when we consider the consequences of its absence.

Supporting Children in Health Systems

Children in the health system can present with and develop many psychosocial and emotional needs. For this text, the health system is recognised as '…all organizations, people, and actions whose primary intent is to promote, restore or maintain health' [8]. Anxiety, depression, pain, sleep disturbances, disruption to schooling, and separation from social groups are just some of the associated concerns in the peri-trauma period [9–11]. Long-term consequences include avoidance of future medical treatment [9], Post Traumatic Stress Symptoms (PTSS), and Paediatric Medical Traumatic Stress (PMTS) [9–18]. The reduction of children's distress and subsequent development of ongoing problems is therefore essential. The complexity of connection between children and family also finds families to be both a source of support and possible risk factors for PTSS and PMTS. Therapeutic interventions should then also consider child and family.

The play in play therapy is a developmentally sensitive and natural form of expression for children's thoughts and emotions, learning, processing of experiences, and way to make sense of their world [19]. Play-based approaches support children's coping ability in hospital settings [20, 21], reduce anxiety [21], offer distraction, procedural preparation, increase medical condition and treatment knowledge [20, 22], enhance communication [23, 24], and support emotional well-being [23], amongst other proven outcomes. Play approaches can also be taught to and used by family members to strengthen family relationships and support children [25].

Although play is used by professionals specifically trained to work with children in health settings, it is important that all involved with children understand how they can also use playful approaches to support the children and families that they encounter. Whilst some aspects of therapy require extensive training, there is much that health professionals can do to ease the fear and anxiety of children and caregivers in relation to hospital and the associated procedures and experiences. Time spent to reduce and prevent medical trauma now can make a lifetime of difference for a child.

Whilst many professionals use play in their work with children, how they use and refer to it, differs. The following is a guide to understanding the different uses of play and play therapy in the health field and the terms that may be encountered. This is followed by a consideration of the importance of play, the origins of plays use in therapy, and an explanation of each of the 20 core Therapeutic Powers of Play. These topics help to situate the use of play and give a foundation as to why we do what we do.

Definitions of Play and Play Therapy in the Health System

The following definitions originate from different professional disciplines. They offer a way to understand terms used and seek to create a common language. Figure 1 displays nurses' perceptions of the different types of play for children in hospital and who could be utilised to offer them. The three categories are identified as normative, educative, and therapeutic play. As it encompasses basic play interventions through to a complexity in knowledge and skills for therapeutic play interventions, the categories are a starting point and should be used with discretion. Understanding the types of play, play therapy, and increasing complexity, along with knowledge of client needs, can support awareness of possible need for referral to appropriately trained and qualified professionals.

Extending on the categories of play, Fig. 2 provides another visual representation of the increasing complexity of knowledge and skills required to use the different forms of play and play therapies. Understanding these, along with knowledge of clients and their needs, can support referrals to appropriately trained and qualified professionals where necessary. To ensure common language for each level of the hourglass and specifically in relation to medical play definitions are expanded on in more detail following the play therapy hourglass graphic.

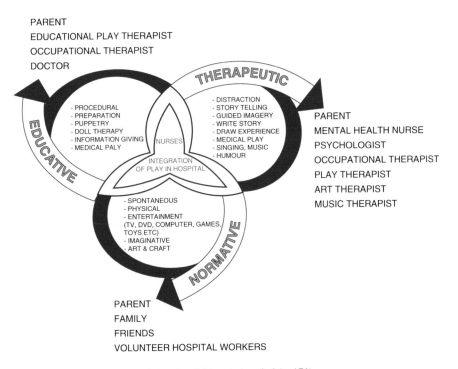

Fig. 1 Parson [1] categories of play for children in hospital (p. 171)

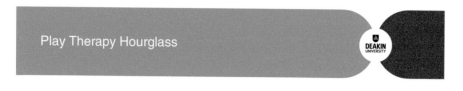

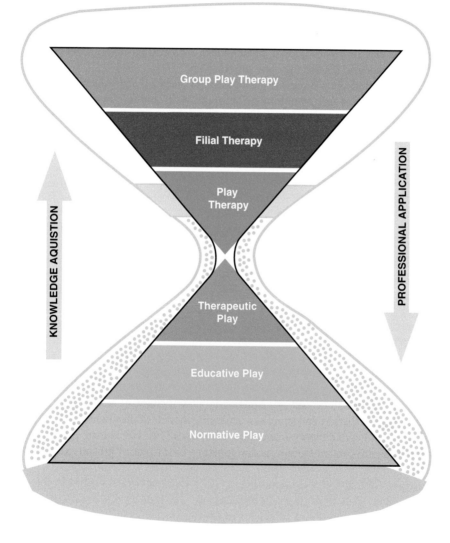

Play Therapy Hourglass

Group Play Therapy

Filial Therapy

Play Therapy

KNOWLEDGE AQUISTION

PROFESSIONAL APPLICATION

Therapeutic Play

Educative Play

Normative Play

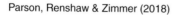

Parson, Renshaw & Zimmer (2018)

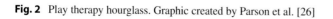

deakin.edu.au/play

Fig. 2 Play therapy hourglass. Graphic created by Parson et al. [26]

Medical play involves 'a medical theme or medical equipment' ([27], p. 9). It helps the child to overcome fear of medical equipment and experiences through familiarisation with basic equipment, art experiences using medical supplies, and acting out medical procedures using toys and role play [2]. As medical play is used in multiple ways, for this chapter the more specific terms 'educative play' and 'therapeutic play' will be used.

Normative play involves the normal play of childhood such as puzzles, games, sports, art, and craft [2]. It helps to make the hospital a more normal environment. Normative play promotes normal development, offers stress relief, supports building of a therapeutic relationship, and provides fun [27].

Educative play is a directive pre-procedural form of play suited to hospitals [28]. It may involve preparation by pre-hospital visits and programmes that orient children to the ward, children's books on hospitalisation, prior demonstration of procedures on dolls/toys, and providing information in a variety of formats to parents.

Therapeutic play may be directive or non-directive [28]. It supports coping and psychosocial wellbeing, and offers preparation for medical procedures [2, 27]. Procedural preparation would be undertaken prior to procedures (educative play), whereas activities to help with expressing emotions, understand a child's thinking, or to help them to cope may be used any time throughout the hospital experience [2, 28].

Play Therapy is practised by trained play therapists who support clients to work through psychological, social, emotional, and behavioural concerns and to enhance development. Whilst there are many play therapy models, a safe environment, play, the Therapeutic Powers of Play (TPoP), and the therapeutic relationship are pivotal components of play therapy in general. Play therapy is a therapeutic approach and Play Therapists require training and education in child development, mental health, play, trauma, neurodevelopmental disorders, counselling skills, amongst other areas.

It is important to acknowledge that within the discipline of Play Therapy, a range of practice models are available that theoretically support clinical practice. For example, psychoanalytic and psychodynamic play therapy, systemic play therapy, humanistic play therapy and some new emerging models of play therapy which may draw on and integrate theory from other disciplines [29]. Humanistic play therapy draws on person-centred therapy as developed by Carl Rogers [30] and extended by Virginia Axline [31] to work with children, she called this Non-Directive Play Therapy (NDPT)and is also referred to as Child-Centred Play Therapy (CCPT). In this approach the therapeutic relationship and the therapeutic qualities of the practitioner provide the conditions for healing and growth.

Axline [31] developed the eight basic principles, which include that the play therapist:

1. Develops a warm, friendly relationship with the child.
2. Accepts the child exactly as they are.
3. Establishes a feeling of permissiveness within the relationship so the child can fully express their thoughts and feelings.

4. Attunes to the child's feelings and reflects these back to help the child gain insight into their behaviour.
5. Respects the child's ability to solve their own problems, leaving responsibility to make choices.
6. Tries not to direct the child's behaviour or conversation, but rather the therapist follows the child's lead.
7. Tries not to attempt to rush therapy and recognises that therapy may be a gradual therapeutic process.
8. Sets only limits that anchor the child to reality or make the child aware of responsibilities in the relations.

Whilst it is not always possible to employ all eight principles in all situations, it is possible to communicate a humanistic attitudinal stance.

Medical Play Therapy uses play therapy approaches to support children with medically related concerns. Psychological issues may develop in relation to a medical (usually chronic) condition, its management, and the resultant impact on life. Food allergies, for example, are associated with anxiety, social fears such as exclusion, avoidance of social activities, eating and nutritional concerns, lower self-esteem, and hypervigilance [32]. Children may have experienced trauma as a result of medical procedures, accidents, injuries, and witnessing a distressing incident, and need help to resolve PTSS or PMTS. The injury or medical procedures may have created physical changes and limitations. Anxiety (e.g. separation anxiety) and social implications may develop. Medical Play Therapy may therefore address complex psychological, emotional, physical, and social issues resulting from the trauma or condition itself and resulting injuries and treatment. It can also support children by preparing them for upcoming procedures through exposure to medical equipment and role play. Pretend play can provide opportunities for control and addressing of fears before the day.

Filial Therapy (FT) is a family therapy that uses play therapy skills to strengthen family relationships. Parents are trained in play therapy skills including structuring, empathic listening, imaginative play, and limit setting [25]. They then hold short regular play sessions individually with each child. Play sessions help caregivers to develop an understanding of their child's emotions and world through their child's eyes. Children can express all emotions and feel acceptance by those that they value most. This understanding and acceptance enhances the caregiver–child relationship. Caregivers can develop effective parenting skills, improve communication, and be more united in their parenting approach.

Chronic medical conditions have a significant impact on the lives of children and families. Hospitalisation, appointments, treatment and possible associated discomfort, ongoing care needs, and other stressors contribute to strain on the family and their relationships. Support and repair of family relationships through interventions such as FT is necessary and important. Seymour [33] suggests the use of an adaption of FT for supporting sibling relationships affected by medical experiences. A travel FT kit can be made for families that experience frequent hospitalisation [25].

However, FT is an involved process that is more suited to training families outside of the hospital environment rather than a quick intervention for an acute need.

Child Life Therapy—Professionals supporting children in hospitals are known as 'Child Life Therapists' in Australia, 'Hospital Play Specialists' in the UK and New Zealand, and 'Child Life Professionals' in the USA, Canada, and other countries. Child Life Therapy (CLT) will be used to refer to the work of all these professionals for this section. CLT seeks to normalise the hospital experience for children, provide preparation for procedures, and offer coping strategies to reduce anxiety and prevent long-term problems for children and families [2, 27]. CLT provides individualised interventions for children and families using normative, educative, and medical play. Professionals help to orient children to the hospital environment, provide support to children and families, train health staff on child development and children's developmental, social, and emotional wellbeing [34].

In summary, this section has briefly defined the various types of play and associate skills for therapeutic play interventions. Understanding the types of play and play therapy in the health care setting can support raising awareness and support referral to appropriately trained and qualified professionals. All health care professionals should be aware of and work within a child's rights framework. The convention of the rights of the child is important for this text. Additionally, the convention of the rights of persons with a disability and particularly Article 7—Children with a disability and Article 25—Health.

United Nations Convention on the Rights of the Child

In 1989, a historical commitment was made by leaders around the world to adopt the United Nations Convention on the Rights of the Child (CRC) which is an international agreement which supports children to be safe and have their rights upheld. Each Article relates to areas which impact children and the below in particular relate to children in a hospital setting. UNISEF Australia (2022) states that it has become the most widely ratified human rights treaty and can be used to transform children's lives from around the globe.

One way to systemically advocate for the rights of the child is to teach medical and health care professionals about playful ways of being with, and communicating with, children in a developmentally sensitive manner. This links directly to the UNCRC Articles 12, 13, and 16 and the right of the child to have a say about what they think should happen, to receive and provide information and the right to have this delivered in privacy [35]. Responding to these Articles in a play-based way ensures that children has their voice heard and can communicate in an age-appropriate way. As stated earlier, play is the way children communicate and may be the most accessible way for the child to receive and offer important information.

Article 12 of the UNCRC rights of the child states: 'Children have the right to say what they think should happen when adults are making decisions that affect them and to have their opinions taken into account'. Gaining a child's assent is therefore a vital component of the UNCRC Rights of the child to consider. Being able to ensure the child understands what will happen to them when they are being assessed is paramount to ensuring the child feels safe and ethical care is provided. Developmentally sensitive play-based ways of working ensure that the child has the best opportunity to understand the process of assessment as well as be offered appropriate choices regarding their care. This may be provided in a show and tell play-based information session so that the child is well prepared for health care encounters.

Providing Atraumatic Care

Atraumatic care is the provision of therapeutic care by health care professionals using interventions that eliminates or at least minimises the psychological and physiological distress experienced by children and their families in the health care system [36]. One way to provide atraumatic care is using therapeutic play. Nurses and health care professionals can address feelings of vulnerability through sensitive and child focused clinical practice which integrates the principles and skills found in play therapy.

> Play therapy, in all its forms, can help to alleviate such stress, and facilitate a smoother adjustment to the new and potentially frightening surroundings. ([37] p. 77).

This text is aimed to introduce a range of therapeutic play strategies and selected play therapy models of practice, which have been used to activate the therapeutic powers of play within the health settings [37, 38] and more specifically in relation to medical play [39] and procedural play associated with invasive procedures [40, 41]. Thus, therapeutic play is useful for children to deal with the clinical aspects of hospital treatment by creating and recreating the child's reality through play.

Play is a crucial part of the child's world in every way, physically, emotionally, psychologically and socially and should be integrated into all aspects of the child's health care experiences. Erik Erikson, an expert in lifespan psychosocial development, defined child's play as an infantile form of human ability to work through experiences by creating or recreating model situations and to master reality through planning and experimenting [42]. The child may play out their thoughts and feelings at any stage of the health care encounter. Therefore, when therapeutic play is integrated it becomes a useful medium to help assess, plan, implement, evaluate, and reflect upon health care practices and optimise healing.

Reflective Questions and Activities

- What are some benefits that play has as a form of therapy?
- Everyone has different ideas of what is play and what they find playful. Explain why it is important to identify individual client's interests and preferences. How can you cater for this in practice?

- Discuss some of the short and long-term consequences for children and families of medical trauma.
- What type of play could facilitate a developmentally appropriate way to help communicate medical information?
- Consider how you would seek child assent.
- Reflect on how you may integrate the UNCRC.

Orientation to the Text

This text is organised into three sections. Part 1, including this chapter, provides the theoretical background and specific definitions that help to contextualise the way health care professionals integrate therapeutic play and play therapy in health care settings. These definitions are important to have a shared discourse in health care settings as play and play therapy have been found to be marginalised if not silenced [43]. In the next chapter, Melita and Parson (Chap. 2) provide further information about the history of play therapy and the therapeutic powers of play with specific attention to the 20 core agents of change [44]. Reid-Searl (Chap. 3) introduces the seven C's of caring which is important to extend the humanistic stance to hospital and health care encounters. Dean, Parson, and Stagnitti (Chap. 4) provide an overview of therapeutic play approaches to allow assessments to be approached in a diverse, creative and developmentally sensitive ways. Hadiprodjo (Chap. 5) finalises this section with important considerations in relation to attachment theory in health care.

In Part 2, the text provides information about the various stages of child development which are useful to consider when working in a child sensitive manner from infancy to adolescence. In this section, the developmental stages are aligned with Erik Erikson's psychosocial stages, play and neurological development. Implications for working with children in each stage of development provides nursing and allied health care professionals with useful insights in communicating in developmentally sensitive ways. Dooley (Chap. 6) explores therapeutic play and maintains hope in the infant child, Breguet (Chap. 7) addresses therapeutic play, volition, and the toddler, Hallowell (Chap. 8) debates therapeutic play and aiding purpose in the preschooler, Hickson (Chap. 9) discusses therapeutic play and instilling competence in the school aged child and finally Godfrey, Dean, and Hadiprodjo (Chap. 10) examine therapeutic play, fidelity, and the teenager.

Clinical case scenarios are presented in part 3 of the text, whereby the authors draw on their clinical experience to integrate how they have used therapeutic play to communicate with children in various health care settings. Perrin (Chap. 11) introduces Jesse who requires preparation for allergy assessment, Sarah (Chap. 12) presents the case study of Evan and his need to be supported whilst experiencing Botox injections for the treatment of cerebral palsy. Renshaw (Chap. 13) showcases how play therapy may be accessed in a community health setting as Connor was struggling to stay at school due to an underlying health concern resulting in encopresis and enuresis. Next, Dean (Chap. 14) discusses Bartholomew and how he learns about his diabetes diagnosis and associated treatment. Butler (Chap. 15) shares her therapeutic work through the eyes of Charlotte and how she was able to integrate child-centred play therapy in a hospice environment. Hadiprodjo, Parson, and Dean (Chap. 16) conclude the book with a final overview summary.

Additional Resources

- United Nations Convention on the rights of the child (UNCRC). https://www.ohchr.org/en/instruments-mechanisms/instruments/convention-rights-child.
- For a simplified version of the UNCRC list visit UNISEF. https://www.unicef.org.au/upload/unicef/media/unicef-simplified-convention-child-rights.pdf.
- United Nations Convention on the rights of persons with a disability (UNCRPD). https://www.ohchr.org/en/instruments-mechanisms/instruments/convention-rights-persons-disabilities.

References

1. Parson, J. (2008) Integration of procedural play for children undergoing cystic fibrosis treatment: a nursing perspective. Unpublished PhD. International Program for Psychosocial Health Research. Central Queensland University.
2. Brown, F., Clark, C. D., & Patte, M. M. (2018). Therapeutic work with children in diverse settings. In L. C. Rubin (Ed.), *Handbook of medical play therapy and child life* (pp. 3–18). Taylor Francis Group.
3. Sutton-Smith, B. (2001). *The ambiguity of play*. Harvard University Press.
4. Landreth, G. L. (2012). *Play therapy: The art of the relationship* (3rd ed.). Routledge.
5. Van den Berg, C. L., Hol, T., Van Ree, J. M., Spruijt, B. M., Everts, H., & Koolhaas, J. M. (1999). Play is indispensable for an adequate development of coping with social challenges in the rat. *Developmental Psychobiology, 34*(2), 129–138.
6. Brown, S. (2014b, June 1). Play deprivation...A leading indicator for mass murder. The National Institute for Play. http://www.nifplay.org/play-deprivation-a-leading-indicator-for-mass-murder/
7. Brown, S. L. (2014a). Consequences of play deprivation. *Scholarpedia, 9*(5), 30449. https://doi.org/10.4249/scholarpedia.30449
8. World Health Organisation (WHO). (2007). *Everybody business: Strengthening health systems to improve health outcomes: WHO's framework for action*. WHO Press. https://www.who.int/healthsystems/strategy/everybodys_business.pdf
9. Ben-Ari, A., Benarroch, F., Sela, Y., & Margalit, D. (2020). Risk factors for the development of medical stress syndrome following surgical intervention. *Journal of Pediatric Surgery, 55*(9), 1685–1690. https://doi.org/10.1016/j.jpedsurg.2019.11.011
10. Christian-Brandt, A. S., Santacrose, D. E., Farnsworth, H. R., & MacDougall, K. A. (2019). When treatment is traumatic: An empirical review of interventions for pediatric medical traumatic stress. *American Journal of Community Psychology, 64*(3), 389–404. https://doi.org/10.1002/ajcp.12392
11. Ramsdell, K. D., Morrison, M., Kassam-Adams, N., & Marsac, M. L. (2016). A qualitative analysis of children's emotional reactions during hospitalization following injury. *Journal of Trauma Nursing, 23*(4), 194–201. https://doi.org/10.1097/JTN.0000000000000217

12. Daviss, W., Mooney, D., Racusin, R., Ford, J., Fleischer, A., & McHugo, G. (2000). Predicting posttraumatic stress after hospitalization for pediatric injury. *Journal of the American Academy of Child & Adolescent Psychiatry, 39*(5), 576–583. https://doi.org/10.1097/00004583-200005000-00011

13. Flaum Hall, M., & Hall, S. E. (2013). When treatment becomes trauma: Defining, preventing, and transforming medical trauma. In Ideas and research you can use: VISTAS 2013. 73. https://www.counseling.org/docs/default-source/vistas/when-treatment-becomes-trauma-defining-preventing-.pdf.

14. Kassam-Adams, N., Marsac, M. L., Hildenbrand, A., & Winston, F. (2013). Posttraumatic stress following pediatric injury: update on diagnosis, risk factors, and intervention. *JAMA Pediatrics, 167*(12), 1158–1165. https://doi.org/10.1001/jamapediatrics.2013.2741

15. Kazak, A. E., Kassam-Adams, N., Schneider, S., Zelikovsky, N., Alderfer, M. A., & Rourke, M. (2006). An integrative model of pediatric medical traumatic stress. *Journal of Pediatric Psychology, 31*(4), 343–355. https://doi.org/10.1093/jpepsy/jsj054

16. Marsac, M. L., Kassam-Adams, N., Delahanty, D., Widaman, K., & Barakat, L. P. (2014). Posttraumatic stress following acute medical trauma in children: a proposed model of biopsycho-social processes during the peri-trauma period. *Clinical Child & Family Psychology Review, 17*(4), 399–411. https://doi.org/10.1007/s10567-014-0174-2

17. Perry, B. D. (2007). *Stress, trauma, and post-traumatic stress disorders in children.* Child Trauma Academy. https://www.complextrauma.ca/wp-content/uploads/C9-PTSD-in-Children-An-Introduction-.pdf

18. Triantafyllou, C., & Matziou, V. (2019). Aggravating factors and assessment tools for posttraumatic stress disorder in children after hospitalization. *Psychiatriki, 30*(3), 256–266. https://doi.org/10.22365/jpsych.2019.303.256

19. Bennett, M. M., & Eberts, S. (2014). Self-expression. In C. E. Schaefer & A. A. Drewes (Eds.), *The therapeutic powers of play: 20 core agents of change* (2nd ed., pp. 11–24). John Wiley & Sons Inc..

20. Gaynard, L., Goldberger, J., & Laudley, L. N. (1991). The use of stuffed, body-outline dolls with hospitalized children and adolescents. *Children's Health Care, 20*(4), 216–224. https://doi.org/10.1207/s15326888chc2004_4

21. Li, W. H. C., Chung, J. O. K., Ho, K. Y., & Kwok, B. M. C. (2016). Play interventions to reduce anxiety and negative emotions in hospitalized children. *BMC Pediatrics, 16*(36). https://doi.org/10.1186/s12887-016-0570-s

22. Gjærde, L. K., Hybschmann, J., Dybdal, D., Topperzer, K. M., SchrØder, M. A., Gibson, J. L., Ramchandani, P., Ginsberg, E. I., Ottesen, B., Frandsen, T. L., & SØrensen, J. L. (2021). Play interventions for paediatric patients in hospital: a scoping review. *BMJ Open, 11*. https://doi.org/10.1136/bmjopen-2021-051957

23. Moerman, C. J., & Jansens, R. M. L. (2020). Using social robot PLEO to enhance the Well-being of hospitalised children. *Journal of Child Health Care, 0*(0), 1–15. https://doi.org/10.1177/1367493520947503

24. Sposito, A. M. P., de Sparapani, B. C., de Lima, R. A. G., Silva-Rodrigues, F. M., Nascimento, L. C., Pfeifer, L. I., & de Montigny, F. (2016). Puppets as a strategy for communication with Brazilian children with cancer. *Nursing and Health Sciences, 18*(1), 30–37. https://doi.org/10.1111/nhs.12222

25. Van Fleet, R. (2018). Family-oriented treatment of childhood chronic medical illness: the power of play in filial therapy. In L. C. Rubin (Ed.), *Handbook of medical play therapy and child life* (pp. 257–276). Taylor Francis Group.

26. Parson, J. A., Renshaw, K. L., & Zimmer, T. (2018). *Play therapy hourglass.* Deakin University.

27. Burns-Nader, S., & Hernandez-Reif, M. (2016). Facilitating play for hospitalized children through child life services. Children's Health Care, 45(1), 1–21. https://doi.org/10.1080/02739615.2014.948161

28. Parson, J. (2003, Nov 13–14). Discovering successful play strategies for children undergoing invasive procedures [Paper presentation]. Central Queensland University Women in Research Conference, Rockhampton, Queensland, Australia. https://acquire.cqu.edu.au/articles/confer-

ence_contribution/Discovering_successful_play_strategies_for_children_undergoing_invasive_procedures/13402148

29. Schaefer, C. E. (2011). *Foundations of play therapy* (2nd ed.). John Wiley & Sons.
30. Rogers, C. R. (1961). *On becoming a person*. Houghton Mifflin.
31. Axline, V. (1947). *Play therapy*. Ballantine.
32. Polloni, L., & Muraro, A. (2020). Anxiety and food allergy: a review of the last two decades. *Clinical and Experimental Allergy: Journal of the British Society for Allergy and Clinical Immunology, 50*(4), 420–441. https://doi.org/10.1111/cea.13548
33. Seymour, J. W. (2018). What about me? Sibling play therapy when a family has a child with chronic illness. In L. C. Rubin (Ed.), *Handbook of medical play therapy and child life* (pp. 237–256). Taylor Francis Group.
34. Association of Child Life Therapists Australia (ACLTA) (2021). *What is Child Life Therapy?* http://childlife.org.au/about-child-life-therapy/what-is-child-life-therapy/
35. Edwards, J., Parson, J., & O'Brien, W. (2016). Child play therapists' understanding and application of the United Nations convention on the rights of the child: a narrative analysis. *International Journal of Play Therapy, 25*(3), 133–145.
36. Hockenberry, M. J., Rodgers, C. C., & Wilson, D. (2022). *Wong's essentials of pediatric nursing* (11th ed.). Elsevier.
37. Doverty, N. (1992). Therapeutic use of play in hospital. *British Journal of Nursing, 1*(2), 77, 79–81.
38. Hall, T. M., Kaduson, H. G., & Schaefer, C. E. (2002). Fifteen effective play therapy techniques. *Professional Psychology Research & Practice, 33*(6), 515–522.
39. Jessee, P. O., Wilson, H., & Morgan, D. (2000). Medical play for young children. *Childhood Education, 76*(4), 215.
40. Favara-Scacco, C., Smirne, G., Schiliro, G., & Di Cataldo, A. (2001). Art therapy as support for children with leukemia during painful procedures. *Medical & Pediatric Oncology, 36*(4), 474–480.
41. Powers, S. W. (1999). Empirically supported treatments in pediatric psychology: procedure-related pain. *Journal of Pediatric Psychology, 24*(2), 131–145.
42. Erikson, E. H. (1963). *Childhood and society* (2nd ed.). Norton.
43. Parson, J. (2017). Caring for children with cystic fibrosis in a hospital setting in Australia the space where play and pain meet. In L. C. Rubin (Ed.), *Handbook of medical play therapy and child life: interventions in clinical and medical settings*. Routledge.
44. Schaefer, C. E., & Drewes, A. A. (2014). *The therapeutic powers of play: 20 core agents of change* (2nd ed.). John Wiley & Sons.

Play in Therapy and the Therapeutic Powers of Play

Fiona M. Melita and Judi A. Parson

Objectives

At the end of this chapter, you will be able to:

- recall at least 3 key scholars who influenced the development of play therapy.
- understand why identifying and using change mechanisms is more important than adhering to a single therapeutic technique.
- identify and consider the Therapeutic Powers of Play for practice in health settings.

Introduction

Although play is used by professionals specifically trained to work with children in health settings, it is important that all involved with children understand how they can also use playful approaches to support the children and families that they encounter. While some aspects of therapy require extensive training, there is much that health professionals can do to ease the fear and anxiety of children and caregivers in relation to hospital and the associated procedures and experiences. Time spent to reduce and prevent medical trauma now can make a lifetime of difference for a child. While many professionals use play in their work with children, how they use and refer to it differs. This chapter explains each of the 20 core Therapeutic Powers of Play which have been identified as the heart and soul of play therapy [1]. Firstly, an overview of the early origins of play therapy.

F. M. Melita (✉)
Becoming Me Play Therapy (BMPT), Townsville, QLD, Australia
e-mail: fiona@becomingmeplaytherapy.com.au

J. A. Parson
School of Health and Social Development, Deakin University, Geelong, VIC, Australia

J. A. Parson et al. (eds.), *Integrating Therapeutic Play Into Nursing and Allied Health Practice*, https://doi.org/10.1007/978-3-031-16938-0_2

Play in Therapy and Play Therapy: Early Origins

Evidence of children's toys and play from many cultures have been found dating back thousands of years [2]. However, the use of play in therapy is a development of recent times. The author H.G. Wells repeated his own childhood play with his children and formalised it into a book in 1911 called *Floor Games* with the "belief that play promoted a framework for expansive and creative ideas in adulthood" [3, p. 2]. Although Wells did not interpret the play or recognise its psychological significance, he took interest in the work of Carl Jung and was forward thinking for his time [3]. *Floor Games* later inspired Margaret Lowenfeld and contributed to child therapy [3].

Dr. Hermine Hug-Hellmuth was the first to practise psychoanalysis with children and to publish papers on play therapy [4]. From 1909 to early her death in 1924 she recognised the influence of play on child development, its importance in understanding the child, used observations and play in sessions, interpreted symbols and content expressed in play, and developed play therapy techniques [4]. Her contribution to children's therapy was large but recognition has been dwarfed by later names.

Melanie Klein, beginning in 1919, worked with children younger than Dr. Hug-Hellmuth. She maintained a free association approach, but recognised toys as children's means of communication [5]. In developing her "psychoanalytic play technique" she discovered plays value in establishing relationships, accessing the unconscious [6], and noted the need for a separate therapy environment rather than using everyday places like the home [5]. It was Klein that began the use of miniatures in therapy, ensuring available choices allowed varied and creative use. Klein proposed that symbols must be interpreted in the context of the child [5]. She incorporated water activities, drawing, painting, pretend play, craft, and expression of emotions with the materials [5].

Anna Freud began in education, later training and practising as a children's psychoanalyst, and first publishing in 1922 [7]. She examined children's play in therapy to understand how they expressed, failed to express, and changed emotions during play [8]. She recognised environmental influences on children and emphasised the importance of the therapeutic relationship in bringing about change [8].

Margaret Lowenfeld was greatly inspired by the play experiences described in H.G. Wells' book, *Floor Games* [9]. From this, she developed the Lowenfeld World Technique which seeks to understand the child's world of feelings and ideas through their creation of miniature worlds in sand [10]. She developed other methods for observing and working with children and gave voice to children without the need for words. Lowenfeld understood the sensory experience and spontaneity of children and so enabled an environment of free expression in which children with difficulties could play while they were supported therapeutically [10]. In this environment, Lowenfeld practised many ideas that exist in current child therapy including but not limited to: positioning to not be above a child, a child-centred environment, rules and limits, and confidentiality [11]. Lowenfeld also believed that the mind and body should not be separated, thereby recognising the wholeness of a person, the importance of culture, and that experiences are subjective [11].

There have been many contributors since to the development of play therapy, but from these early origins we can recognise many of the ideas and practices that exist in the different play therapy models of today. What has progressed substantially since these early times is the understanding in what creates change for clients. While early therapists disagreed with the theoretical approach of others and held firmly to their own, recognition continues to grow that there are common factors between approaches. These factors create the change for clients and identifying and understanding them is more important and allows for greater flexibility in meeting client needs. The next section looks at the factors that have been identified in play as "change agents" for clients.

The Therapeutic Powers of Play: Mechanisms of Change

Kazdin [12] proposes that there are likely common change mechanisms amongst the many existing therapies and identification and focus on these would better address the needs of clients. In play, 20 factors (Fig. 1) or "change mechanisms" have been identified by Schaefer and Drewes [13]. These increased from the 14 initially identified by Charles Schaefer in 1993 which he named the "Therapeutic Powers of Play" (TPoP) [14]. The TPoP are categorised into four sections; *Facilitates Communication*, *Fosters Emotional Wellness*, *Enhances Social Relationships*, and *Increases Personal Strengths*. Use of the TPoP enables selection of the appropriate change agents for each client to create individual treatment plans as opposed to a single play therapy model approach [15]. Understanding why we use and what we use and choosing appropriately for each client is essential [12]. The remainder of this chapter explains each therapeutic power and is followed by a clinical example to demonstrate their use.

Self-Expression

Play is its own language. Through play, an intensity and depth can be expressed that for many reasons, is not possible through words. Without the complex spoken language and abstract thinking of those older, younger children can share their view of the world through play [13]. Even when children do not feel comfortable to talk, the unconscious world naturally appears in play, giving insight to their thoughts and concerns. For some, it is easier to depict creatively than in words. Play gives the freedom to be or do anything and so explore experiences, fears, and ideas safely.

Access to the Unconscious

The implicit memories of early childhood, while not consciously recalled, continue to affect throughout life. Emotions can also occur outside of conscious awareness and affect behaviour and reactions [16]. Through symbolism, play affords distance

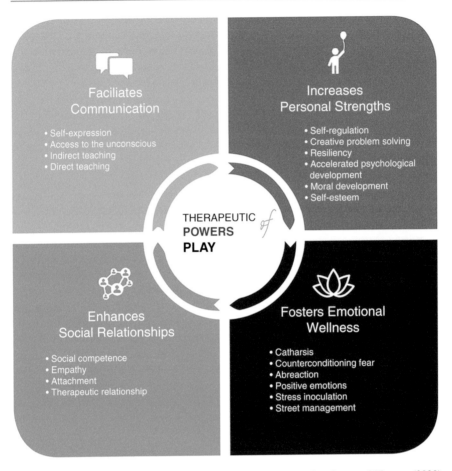

Fig. 1 The therapeutic powers of play. Graphic created by Parson, Renshaw, and Zimmer (2020) adapted from Schaefer and Drewes [13]. The therapeutic powers of play: 20 core agents of change (second ed.). NJ: John Wiley & Sons

from uncomfortable and distressing material and a way to connect with unrecognised emotions. Symbols can represent an item, concept, relationship, place, action, or idea. Early memories, unconscious emotions, and concerns that are difficult or not possible to verbalise, can be brought to light and worked through in play [15]. Expressive experiences such as art and play directly engage with the unconscious and implicit memories.

Direct Teaching

Direct teaching uses "instruction, modelling, guided practice, and positive reinforcement" ([17], p. 43) to learn new things and practise skills. Play is fun and with most children's natural inclination to play, it makes it an ideal medium for learning.

Even for adults, when an experience is enjoyable, we are motivated to join in and want to continue. Learning through play allows active involvement, repetition for consolidation, modelling, and enjoyment. Children can be fully immersed in the experience and play, and materials can be targeted to the individual child's interest, thereby ensuring to capture attention and provide motivation.

Indirect Teaching

Indirect methods are used to guide, teach, connect emotionally or through a relatable experience, and create distance from difficult content. An indirect approach can reduce resistance and allow issues to be faced in a less threatening way [15]. Stories (bibliotherapy), art, puppets, sand tray, metaphor [18], and other playful activities may be used. Resistance is the difficulty someone is having in facing their struggles or in the work they need to do. Indirect teaching methods can support the client by offering a safety and distance that afford greater tolerance to approach difficult content. For example, children may be read stories about a child with similar problems, which allows them to connect with the character and understand their situation, empathise, change their behaviour, problem solve something in their life, understand others, or recognise that others feel that way too and not feel so alone. This can be more comfortable than having to sit and talk about their problems with someone.

Catharsis

Catharsis refers to the release of strong emotions that can bring about positive change and closure. Jackson [19] explains that release occurs in conjunction with remembering of a traumatic or distressing experience. Catharsis is often also associated with cognitive processing and the development of insight [20]. It requires a safe environment and can be brought about through a variety of techniques such as music, play, drama, art, writing, sand tray, talking, and physical exercise.

Abreaction

Abreaction involves the release of previously inhibited emotions. Emotions may have been withheld or prevented from being expressed at the time of the trauma. In "abreactive play", replaying of the experience helps to bring it to conscious awareness where the individual can have control, release appropriate emotions, and hopefully process and resolve the trauma in the safety of a therapeutic relationship, thereby creating a coherent narrative [15]. The emotions can then be paired with the experience, preventing their continued presentation from the unconscious into consciousness and subsequent disruption of present-day life [15]. In play, the individual can work through a frightening or stressful experience at a distance through symbolic materials such as miniatures and without the need to talk. Play being non-verbal also allows for processing of unconscious early trauma. Abreaction and catharsis are intricately linked; however, abreaction typically refers to just the emotional release [19].

Positive Emotions

Positive emotions enable steps of positive growth. In moments of positivity, we can find clarity that may have been blocked in the presence of negative emotions. This clarity can allow us insight into problems, to "contemplate new ideas, develop alternative solutions, reinterpret their situations, reflect on behaviors, and initiate new courses of action and creative endeavours" [21, p. 139]. A study by Brockington et al. [22] found that storytelling with children in hospital intensive care units produced benefits including significant reductions in pain scores and cortisol levels, and increased oxytocin levels. Cortisol is a hormone associated with stress. Oxytocin is related to many functions but is linked with empathy and emotional processing [22]. Play itself is enjoyable for children and lends itself to the elicitation of positive emotions and experiences. Additionally, the opportunities for learning, growth, and development that play offers in this environment of positive emotions demonstrate plays' dual value.

Counterconditioning of Fears

Counterconditioning is the reduction or elimination of negative responses to stressful and anxiety provoking stimuli. Usually, an experience that elicits an opposing response is paired with the fear-provoking stimuli in order to reduce the level of reactivity [23]. With repetition of this over time, the fear is reduced. A young child may be offered a playful game, while older children and adults may be taught a specific opposing response such as relaxation to use [23].

Stress Inoculation

Stress inoculation prepares for situations that induce stress, anxiety, and fear. When given the opportunity to experience something fearful in small amounts or prior to the actual event, the exposure can help to lessen the distress [24]. People can then gain mastery over their emotions and learn strategies to cope when they are presented with situations that they find difficult [24]. With real materials or toys, clients can play out or role-play what will be experienced in a future stressful experience. This will familiarise them with the experience and place them in a position of power where they can work through and master their emotions safely in a situation that they can control. In the case of medical equipment and medical procedures, they can practise undergoing them and so understand what they will have done, become familiar with equipment that will be used, ask questions, and develop coping skills.

Stress Management

Stress is a feeling of psychological, physical, or emotional pressure that the individual feels unable to cope with. Stress is subjective and as such, depends on individual coping, resources, and the interpretation of a situation. The effects of stress on the body are varied, ranging from altered brain development in young children and memory impairments [25] to "cold and respiratory symptoms", "immunologic deficits", "other infections", "heart disease", "sleep-wake cycle disturbances" [26], "heart attacks, arrhythmias, sudden death", "burnout, anxiety disorders, and depression", "diabetes, hair loss, hyperthyroidism, obesity, sexual dysfunction, tooth and gum disease, and ulcers" [27], to name a few.

Stress management involves the development of coping strategies to use with stress and stressful situations. There are many factors that contribute to stress: "age, socioeconomic status, gender, social support status, personality, self-esteem, genetics, life events, experiences, and current health status" [26]. While some of these cannot be changed or avoided, there are effective coping strategies that can be learnt to help prevent and reduce the impact of life stressors [26].

For children, stress management interventions must consider their cognitive development level [28]. Play affords many stress reduction benefits including self-soothing and regulatory opportunities through sand, water, and other sensory materials [28], escape through fantasy and games, or the acting out of difficulties to explore solutions [15]. Directive techniques such as sand trays, breathing exercises, art exercises, and music and relaxation activities can be offered. In the hospital environment, clown doctors have been used to offer the positive benefits of humour, distraction, fun, a "sense of control", and "decrease in negative mood", which has positive benefits for children, caregivers, and staff [29].

Therapeutic Relationship

Landreth [30] considers the therapeutic relationship a shared experience where the client is "fully accepted as a person of worth" through respect, without expectation, and is felt by both the therapist and child. The therapeutic relationship is important for every client and is essential for change. It requires attunement and caring by the therapist. Client's problems may also have developed in or due to relationships and need repair through relationship.

Attachment

Attachment is the bond between an infant and caregiver that develops regardless of the quality of the relationship. However, the quality of the attachment can affect the child's competence and possible development of psychopathology across the lifespan. Secure attachments develop when infants can depend on the caregiver to consistently meet their needs and is associated with better outcomes [31]. Insecure attachments develop when a caregiver does not meet or is inconsistent in meeting a child's needs, which creates stress and activates the fear system [31]. However, attachment is not fixed and experiences through life can alter attachment styles [32].

Attachment changes in adolescence as they go through a process of exploration and mastery [33]. Independence creates less reliance on caregivers and peer relationships take on increasing prominence. While caregivers maintain their place as the primary attachment relationship, when distress is high, peers become sources of attachment as they are sought for support, socialising, and other needs [33]. Adolescents operate from and are influenced by an integration of their earlier attachment experiences, but peer attachments do not have all the qualities of attachment "relationships" [33].

Supporting a child in the therapeutic space to develop a secure attachment can inhibit the fear response and allow them to explore and play with greater ease. Through play, the child can develop skills, grow socially and emotionally, and process difficulties and concerns. Awareness of a child's history and current relationships helps to understand them and their attachments [32]. Awareness of your own attachment history helps to understand your relationship behaviour.

Social Competence

Social competence incorporates those behaviours that are more desirable or "socially acceptable" and as such, allow the individual to engage successfully in the social world. In typical development, social competence improves as children move through developmental stages and interact with others socially and through play. Neurodivergent individuals (Autism, Attention Deficit Hyperactivity Disorder (ADHD), and other) and those with other concerns (e.g. anxiety) may have or develop social skill deficits due to decreased social opportunities or behaviours that negatively affect social interactions [34]. In the long term, those with social skill deficits struggle with friendship, loneliness, and ongoing social difficulties [35]. Games, rough and tumble play, socio-dramatic play, role-playing, and therapeutic storytelling enable children to interact, cooperate, practise, negotiate, face fears, and so develop many social skills [35]. The improvement of pretend play skills in children with these deficits has been shown to contribute to social competence [34], thereby reinforcing the importance of pretend play.

Empathy

Empathy is physically felt, and cognitive and emotional aspects allow us to truly connect with and understand another in a way that enables us to respond appropriately to their feelings and thoughts [36]. This is an important distinction from sympathy, in which similar feelings are aroused because we have experienced something similar. With empathy, we have stepped into the other's experience, from their perspective. We are not thinking about our own similar experience. We are with them in that moment, appraising what it may feel like for them. Empathy also involves communication of that felt connection and understanding [36].

While impairments in empathy are associated with autism and various psychopathologies, impairment can present in anyone, and the level of empathy varies from person to person. Empathy incorporates the individual components "theory of mind, perspective taking, emotional contagion, and affective empathy" [37, p. 141]. Determining which components or if all are affected, distinguishes the different conditions.

Creative Problem Solving

Creative problem solving is associated with coping and adjustment [38]. Pretend play supports creative problem solving as children explore perspectives through different roles and characters, add problems and find alternative solutions. In play they are directly solving problems in creative ways. These engagements in pretence promote the development of divergent thinking; flexibility of thinking and in different directions [39]. Pretend play also enables the reworking of concerns through to resolution. Role-play and puppet play can introduce and provide practice of experiences that elicit strong emotions, which can alleviate anxiety and distress. Russ [39] states that "Affect is intertwined with pretend play". Positive emotions, child-led play, a safe environment, and a strong therapeutic relationship can all support creative problem solving by lowering defences to allow the freedom to expand thinking and creativity.

Resiliency

Resiliency is the ability to withstand and recover from adversity. Grotberg [40] identified 15 resilience factors related to children that stem from external, internal, and interpersonal sources. The resilience factors that pertain to play therapy and play include trusting relationships, structure and limits, autonomy, "sense of being lovable", self-esteem, locus of control, communication, problem solving, and impulse control [40]. Play therapy offers this through unconditional positive regard, the therapeutic relationship, therapeutic limits, enabling non-verbal and verbal means of communication, responsibility for self, and its child-led and child-paced nature [30]. In play and pretend play, children create problems, devise varied solutions, learn to regulate emotions, develop self-control, and experience autonomy, all of which have been found to promote resilience in children [40]. Given the right conditions, children "possess an innate capacity to strive toward growth and maturity" [30, p. 48]. These conditions exist within the play therapy relationship [30].

Moral Development

Piaget recognises that the development of cognition and morality are linked and that with each, children experience phases rather than stages [41]. Social experiences and culture also play parts in the shaping of moral development. As thinking becomes more complex, moral development advances; a concept also supported by Kohlberg's research (Handy Answer, 2016). The young child's "moral absolutism" of right and wrong and adult authority, progresses to the "moral relativism" of the older child with more flexible thoughts, consideration of multiple viewpoints, emotions, rights, justice, and the possibility to change rules [41].

Accelerated Psychological Development

Psychological development incorporates cognitive, social, emotional, and physical development and occurs in relationship with others. Children are naturally motivated to play, and play can provide experiences that support each of these areas. As play can allow children to do, be, and try almost anything, it can move them to achieve greater than they would in everyday life. Vygotsky [42] proposes a "zone of proximal development", which is the difference between what someone can do with support but are not quite ready to achieve without it. When we watch children take on adult roles, face fears, and persevere at difficult tasks in play, it is easy to understand how play can accelerate children's psychological development.

Self-Regulation

Self-regulation is the ability to adapt to social situations and stressors cognitively and emotionally as they arise. The process moves from external to internal control from infancy through childhood and is then challenged again during the pubertal changes in adolescence [43]. Poor regulation is associated with psychological difficulties [43] and an "excess of self-control" has been proposed by some as the cause of some psychological concerns ([44], p. 177). Berger [43] identifies "attention" as important in self-regulation and its associated factors: "inhibitory control, strategies of problem solving, and self-monitoring". These features are present in play, placing it well to support the development of self-regulation. Games can involve inhibiting certain behaviours in favour of others (e.g. impulsive actions), and promote rapid attention changes, focused attention, and problem solving. In imaginative play and role-play, children solve problems and play becomes increasingly complex and cooperative through developmental periods. Regulating emotions and behaviour is necessary for children to "stay in the play" and be accepted by others into play.

Self-Esteem

Self-esteem incorporates self-worth and self-concept, considering the personal value or worth that we give to ourselves. What is our self-worth? Do we feel good enough? Could someone love us? Are we worthy a person? Self-concept is complex but relates to the way that we view our unique abilities, behaviours, and other aspects. Our self-esteem can be high or low depending on whether we view ourselves positively or negatively. Self-esteem is ever changing and is affected by environmental and social factors [45]. In play therapy the client enters an environment supportive of positive self-esteem through complete acceptance without judgement, freedom in choice, designed to support growth and empowerment. Through play they can then master difficulties and emotions, experience power and control, and try things they do not feel able to do in the everyday.

When thinking clinically about using the Therapeutic Powers of Play, the more powers that are activated, the more chance there is of effective therapeutic benefit. Change mechanisms are not necessarily effective in isolation and those listed are not exhaustive of the powers that play can offer. For these reasons, familiarity and understanding of the TPoP are encouraged to make them readily accessible and able to be applied naturally when interacting with children and families.

Conclusion

This chapter explored the development of play in therapy as a lead into current thinking that there can be common change mechanisms amongst therapies. By understanding the therapeutic powers of play, clinicians in the health field can have greater awareness of how they can support children and families through play and playful interactions and reduce the impact of medical interventions and medical and hospital experiences. This is particularly relevant in relation to understanding the impact of medical interventions and medical trauma on children.

Reflective Questions and Activities

- How would you engage a child in play to elicit medical themes?
- An adolescent has an extended hospital stay and is confined to their room. They frequently express that they are "bored" and missing friends. What type of play is appropriate to offer, who is best to provide it, and how can you meet their social needs?
- What are six of the specific Therapeutic Powers of Play that relate particularly to children and adolescents in the health system? Discuss how you could use or support their use by children and families.
- Why would it be more important to identify and understand "change mechanisms" in therapies rather than to just learn a therapy technique?
- The importance of the therapeutic relationship has been explained and mentioned many times. What do you currently do to develop a relationship with the children and families you work with? Having more awareness as to its therapeutic value in so many areas for children and how connected the emotional and psychological wellbeing of children and families are, what would you do more of or differently now?

Additional Resources

- Allison, L., & Campbell, C. (2021). *Through a child's eyes: Anna freud's vision.* Anna Freud National Centre for Children and Families. https://www.annafreud. org/insights/blogs/2021/12/through-a-child-s-eyes-anna-freud-s-vision/
- Brown, S. (2018). *Play deprivation can damage early child development.* Child and Family Blog. https://childandfamilyblog.com/play-deprivation-early-child-development/
- Circle of Security International. (2019). *What is the circle of security? Developing specific relationship capacities.* https://www.circleofsecurityinternational.com/circle-of-security-model/what-is-the-circle-of-security/
- Matthews, M., & Silk, G. (2015, February 15). *Calico dolls – A process of play – resource.* The Association for the Wellbeing of Children (AWCH). https://awch. org.au/tag/trauma-dolls/
- Perry, B. (n.d.). *The three r's: Reaching the learning brain.* Beacon House. https://beaconhouse.org.uk/wp-content/uploads/2019/09/The-Three-Rs.pdf
- VanFleet, R. (2010). *Helping children and families through traumatic events.* Family enhancement and play therapy center. http://play-therapy.com/professionals.html#trauma

References

1. Peabody, M. A., & Schaefer, C. E. (2019) The therapeutic powers of play: The heart and soul of play therapy. *PlayTherapy Magazine.* September. (pp. 3–7). A4PT.
2. Renshaw, K. L., & Parson, J. A. (2021). It's a small world: Projective play. In E. Prendiville & J. A. Parson (Eds.), *Clinical applications of the therapeutic powers of play : Case studies in child and adolescent psychotherapy* (pp. 73–86). Taylor & Francis Group.
3. Friedman, H. S., & Mitchell, R. R. (2002). *Sandplay: Past, present and future.* Routledge.
4. MacLean, G. (1986). A brief story about Dr. Hermine hug-Hellmuth. *Canadian Journal of Psychiatry. Revue Canadienne de Psychiatrie, 31*(6), 586–589. https://doi. org/10.1177/070674378603100618
5. Klein, M. (1955). The psychoanalytic play technique. *The American Journal of Orthopsychiatry, 25*(2), 223–237. https://doi.org/10.1111/j.1939-0025.1955.tb00131.x
6. Britzman, D. P. (2016). *Melanie Klein: Early analysis, play, and the question of freedom.* Springer.
7. Ramsden, S. (1982). Anna freud C.B.E. 1885-1982: An appreciation. *Journal of Child Psychotherapy, 8*(2), 113–115. https://doi.org/10.1080/00754178208256761
8. Edgcumbe, R. (2000). *Anna Freud: A view of development, disturbance and therapeutic techniques.* Routledge.
9. Urwin, C. (2005). Introduction. In C. Urwin & J. Hood-Williams (Eds.), *Child psychotherapy, war, and the normal child: Selected papers of Margaret Lowenfeld.* Sussex Academic Press.
10. Toys for Reading a Child's Mind. (1969). *World Medicine., 4*(14), 15–20.
11. Woodcock, T. (n.d.). Guidelines on the therapeutic setting. Author.
12. Kazdin, A. E. (2007). Mediators and mechanisms of change in psychotherapy research. *Annual Review of Clinical Psychotherapy, 2,* 1–27. https://doi.org/10.1146/annurev. clinpsy.3.0.22806.091432

13. Schaefer, C. E., & Drewes, A. A. (2014). *The therapeutic powers of play: 20 core agents of change* (2nd ed.). John Wiley & Sons.
14. Parson, J. A. (2021). Children speak play: Landscaping the therapeutic powers of play. In E. Prendiville & J. A. Parson (Eds.), *Clinical applications of the therapeutic powers of play: Case studies in child and adolescent psychotherapy* (pp. 3–11). Taylor & Francis Group.
15. Drewes, A. A., & Schaefer, C. E. (2016). The therapeutic powers of play. In K. J. O'Connor, C. E. Schaefer, & L. D. Braverman (Eds.), *Handbook of play therapy* (2nd ed., pp. 35–60). John Wiley & Sons.
16. Winkielman, P., & Berridge, K. C. (2004). Unconscious emotion. *American Psychological Society, 13*(3) https://sites.lsa.umich.edu/berridge-lab/wp-content/uploads/sites/743/2019/10/Winkielman-Berridge-Current-Directions-unconscious-emotion-2004-1.pdf
17. Fraser, T. (2014). Direct teaching. In C. E. Schaefer & A. A. Drewes (Eds.), *The therapeutic powers of play: 20 core agents of change* (2nd ed., pp. 39–50). John Wiley & Sons.
18. Ginns-Gruenberg, D., & Bridgman, C. (2021). Using bibliotherapy as a catalyst for change. In G. Kaduson & C. E. Schaefer (Eds.), *Play therapy with children: Modalities for change* (pp. 75–92) https://doi.org/10.1037/0000217-006
19. Jackson, S. W. (1994). Catharsis and abreaction in the history of psychological healing. *Psychiatric Clinics of North America, 17*(3), 471–491.
20. Longe, J. L. (2016). Catharsis. In *Gale encyclopedia of psychology* (3rd ed.) https://search.credoreference.com/content/entry/galegp/catharsis/0
21. Fitzpatrick, M. R., & Stalikas, A. (2008). Positive emotions as generators of therapeutic change. *Journal of Psychotherapy Integration, 18*(2), 137–154. https://doi.org/10.1037/1053-0479.18.2.137
22. Brockington, G., Gomes Moreira, A. P., Stephani Buso, M., Gomes da Silva, S., Altszyler, E., Fischer, R., & Moll, J. (2021). Storytelling increases oxytocin and positive emotions and decreases cortisol and pain in hospitalized children. *Proceedings of the National Academy of Sciences of the United States of America, 118*(22), 1–7. https://doi.org/10.1073/pnas.2018409118
23. Van Hollander, T. (2014). Counterconditioning fears. In C. E. Schaefer & A. A. Drewes (Eds.), *The therapeutic powers of play: 20 core agents of change* (2nd ed., pp. 121–130). John Wiley & Sons.
24. Maag, J. W., & Kotlash, J. (1994). Review of stress inoculation training with children and adolescents: Issues and recommendations. *Behavior Modification, 18*(4), 443–469. https://doi.org/10.1177/01454455940184004
25. Davies, D. (2011). *Child development: A practitioner's guide* (3rd ed.). The Guildford Press.
26. McCance, K. L., & Huether, S. E. (2002). *Pathophysiology: The biologic basis for disease in adults & children* (4th ed.). Mosby.
27. Scott, E. (2020, August 3). *What is stress?* Very Well Mind. https://www.verywellmind.com/stress-and-health-3145086
28. Bemis, K. S. (2014). Stress management. In C. E. Schaefer & A. A. Drewes (Eds.), *The therapeutic powers of play: 20 core agents of change* (2nd ed., pp. 143–153). John Wiley & Sons.
29. Ford, K., Courtney-Pratt, H., Tesch, L., & Johnson, C. (2014). More than just clowns – Clown doctor rounds and their impact for children, families, and staff. *Journal of Child Health Care, 18*(3), 286–296. https://doi.org/10.1177/1367493513490447
30. Landreth, G. L. (2012). *Play therapy: The art of the relationship* (3rd ed.). Routledge.
31. Cassidy, J. (2016). The nature of the child's ties. In J. Cassidy & P. R. Shaver (Eds.), *Handbook of attachment: Theory, research, and clinical applications* (3rd ed., pp. 3–24). Guilford Press.
32. Whelan, W. F., & Stewart, A. L. (2014). Attachment. In C. E. Schaefer & A. A. Drewes (Eds.), *The therapeutic powers of play: 20 core agents of change* (2nd ed., pp. 171–183). John Wiley & Sons.
33. Allen, J. P., & Tan, J. S. (2016). The multiple facets of attachment in adolescence. In J. Cassidy & P. R. Shaver (Eds.), *Handbook of attachment : Theory, research, and clinical applications* (3rd ed., pp. 399–415). Guilford Press.

34. Stagnitti, K., O'Connor, C., & Sheppard, L. (2012). Impact of the learn to play program on play, social competence and language for children aged 5-8 years who attend a specialist school. *Australian Occupational Therapy Journal, 59*(4), 302–311. https://doi.org/10.1111/j.1440-1630.2012.01018.x

35. Nash, J. B. (2014). Social competence. In C. E. Schaefer & A. A. Drewes (Eds.), *The therapeutic powers of play: 20 core agents of change* (2nd ed., pp. 185–193). John Wiley & Sons.

36. Howe, D. (2013). *Empathy: What it is and why it matters.* Palgrave Macmillan.

37. Maibom, H. L. (2020). *Empathy.* Routledge.

38. Eschenbeck, H., Schmid, S., Schröder, I., Wasserfall, N., & Kohlmann, C. W. (2018). Development of coping strategies from childhood to adolescence: Cross-sectional and longitudinal trends. *Zeitschrift Fur Gesundheitspsychologie, 25*(1), 18–30. https://doi.org/10.1027/2512-8442/a000005

39. Russ, S. W. (1998). Play, creativity, and adaptive functioning: Implications for play interventions. *Journal of Clinical Child Psychology, 27*(4), 469–480. https://doi.org/10.1207/s15374424jccp2704_11

40. Grotberg, E. H. (1995). *The international resilience project: Research and application.* Civitan International. https://files.eric.ed.gov/fulltext/ED423955.pdf

41. Vozzola, E. C. (2014). *Moral development: Theory and applications.* Routledge.

42. Vygotsky, L. S. (2021). *L.s. vygotsky's pedological works. Volume 2: The problem of age.* Springer.

43. Berger, A. (2011). *Self-regulation: Brain, cognition, and development.* American Psychological Association.

44. Baumeister, R. F. (2018). *Self-regulation and self-control: Selected works of Roy F. Baumeister.* Routledge.

45. Frey, D. (2014). Self-Esteem. In C. E. Schaefer & A. A. Drewes (Eds.), *The therapeutic powers of play: 20 core agents of change* (2nd ed., pp. 295–318). John Wiley & Sons.

Caring for Children, Families, and Health Care Professionals

Kerry Reid-Searl

Objectives

At the end of this chapter, you will be able to:

- Identify the seven C's of caring and understand how these relate to managing a paediatric patient.
- Gain an insight into the value of self-reflection to appreciate personal attitudes towards play and being a playful practitioner.
- Appreciate a range of strategies for implementing therapeutic play as a health care professional.

Introduction

I open this chapter with a declaration that I write through the experience of a nurse of 35 years and not a play therapist or any other allied health professional. My experience comes from engaging in play not analysing the child at play. I believe I have provided opportunities that have prompted children to explore, investigate, and create whilst in the context of a paediatric ward. My intention has been to provide distractions and create a degree of normality for a child in an unfamiliar setting.

I begin by recalling my time as a nursing student and my favourite placement was children's ward. Being placed in children's ward implied permission to not only watch children play, but also to provide resources to facilitate play and use play as

K. Reid-Searl (✉)
University of Tasmania, Hobart, TAS, Australia

CQUniversity, Norman Gardens, QLD, Australia

Monash University, Melbourne, VIC, Australia
e-mail: kerry.reidseal@utas.edu.au, k.reid-searl@cqu.edu.au

J. A. Parson et al. (eds.), *Integrating Therapeutic Play Into Nursing and Allied Health Practice*, https://doi.org/10.1007/978-3-031-16938-0_3

a strategy to help a child through a procedure, albeit distraction or education. I reflect on how I engaged with the child by using my therapeutic self as a playful practitioner. This was in stark contrast to what I remember as a child in hospital. My first experience was as a six-year-old having a tonsillectomy. This was the same year that my father had died, and I felt stressed about being separated from my mother and my twin sister. It was not usual for parents to stay with their children in hospital, so when my mother left, I remember putting on a plastic pair of sunglasses and crying for a long period. The sounds were unfamiliar, the faces unknown and the smell was nothing like I had ever experienced. I remember lying in bed and wetting myself because the bed was too high for me to get out. There was no night light and nor do I recall a buzzer to call for a nurse. I remember being reprimanded for wetting the bed and having to take off my clothes and get into a hospital bath in front of the nurse. I remember being held firmly for an injection and the big words that the doctors and nurses used that made no sense to me. I do not remember anyone playing with me nor do I recall resources for play. These memories are still with me today.

As I reflect, keywords stand out including anxiety, unfamiliar environment, fear, pain, and coldness. These words are etched in my mind and influence how I practise today. In my role as a nurse, I try to empathize with every child and consider the journey that they are experiencing. I realize it is not possible to understand every child's situation, but to gain some insight into their situation and most importantly establish a therapeutic relationship to facilitate trust is paramount. To achieve this, it is necessary to gain insight into the elements of care and have an appreciation of the value of personal reflection to recognize the value of play.

Attributes of Caring for the Hospitalized Paediatric Patient: A Nurse's Perspective

For children, hospitalization can be a traumatic experience. How the child manages and copes through the experience will be influenced by the health care professional assigned to care for the child and their family. Caring is the art and science of many health care professions. For nursing, it is the foundation of the profession and is encompassed in all that the nurse does. This includes the way the nurse communicates with the child and their family portraying empathy, clarity, appropriate language, kindness, respect, and being an advocate. Caring is also included in the way the nurse undertakes skills including caring to understand what best practice they are performing, caring to explain to the child what is happening and caring to consider the developmental age and temperament of the child to explain procedures or implement strategies around play or distraction.

The attributes of caring as developed by Roach [1–3] include compassion, competence, conscience, confidence, commitment, compartment, and creativity.

The 7 C's of Caring

Compassion

Compassion is about recognizing the emotional state of others and to act to be able to help that person when necessary. In a child's world the impact of being hospitalized may be related to the physical or psychosocial condition they are experiencing, the fear of the unknown, a foreign environment, and the separation from loved ones. To be compassionate requires the health care professional to be empathetic, that is to walk in the shoes of the child and see the experience through their eyes and to be sensitive to their situation [2]. Being compassionate and empathetic also means being aware of any personal bias and judgment because health care professionals caring for children will encounter many different parenting styles and children's responses to events. So how does the health care professional gain insight into what the child might be experiencing to show compassion?

> **Activity**
> *Reflect on your own childhood. Was there a time that you were hospitalized yourself or visited someone else in hospital? If so, what interactions did you have, and did they evoke a feeling of fear? Was there a compassionate person that helped you in this situation?*

Based on your own experience consider looking through the eyes of a child in hospital. Try walking their journey. Sometimes in the busyness in our everyday roles as health care professionals it is possible to lose sight of what that child may be experiencing. The following acronym provides a memory prompt for being empathetic.

Tips in empathy

- **E**motional support.
- **M**anage you own emotions.
- **P**ut yourself in the child's shoes.
- **A**cknowledge what the child is feeling/saying/doing.
- **T**alk to the child with care, concern, and curiosity.
- **H**old the unknown including any assumptions, judgements, or biases.
- **Y**earning is a response to a particular need within the context of the child's situation—can you or someone else meet their yearning needs.

A gentle voice, a kind word, a hand, or a playful gesture can have a positive impact, for not only the child but their caregiver too.

Competence

Competence is about having the required knowledge and skill set to deliver the care. Health care professionals are educated to deliver quality care that is evidence based. The education is ongoing, and the competent health care professional is aware of their own strengths and practice gaps through reflection. They have the skills to acquire knowledge to ensure competency remains. Consider the nurse as the health care professional caring for the 4-month-old infant with respiratory condition such as bronchiolitis. The mother is with her baby and extremely concerned. It is the competent nurse who understands the infant's condition, who monitors the infant accurately, who implements nursing strategies that portray to the caregiver confidence and safe practice. This caregiver will not refer to that nurse as the one who is undertaking regular vital signs, or titrating oxygen to manage the infant's work of breathing and monitoring oxygen saturations, instead they will talk about the kind nurse who provided care in a safe, prompt, and efficient manner.

Conscience

Conscience is about an individual's moral sense of right and wrong and is considered a guide to one's behaviour. Health care professionals are bound by professional standards which inform their conscience about the way they deliver care. This includes making ethical, legal, and moral decisions. Conscience also helps drive health care professionals to increase their knowledge about the care they deliver so that they continue to be competent, accountable, and responsible. Consider the health care professionals caring for a child who has a condition that they are unfamiliar with. The conscience driven health care professional will be aware of his/her responsibility to deliver competent care and will also recognize their own gaps in knowledge and practice. As such they would seek direction and support and take time to gain the necessary knowledge to provide the best quality care.

> **Activity**
> *Reflect on an episode of care that you have been asked to provide which has made you uncomfortable due to a lack of knowledge. How did your conscience guide you in the decisions you made about the delivery of care?*

Confidence

Confidence is about feeling sure of yourself and your abilities as a health care professional to deliver care. Being confident is having the insight to know that you can deliver care, and this comes from having both the knowledge and experience. Being confident is necessary to play the roles required of you as the health care professional. Being confident is important for the child to feel safe in your hands but also their significant other. Your peers will also learn from you. Being confident is also recognizing when you need to seek support from others and speak up.

Activity
Reflect on an episode of care where you felt confident. How did your confidence manifest in your performance? What empowered you with confidence?

Commitment

Commitment is about being dedicated to the cause. As a health professional you are committed to your role. For example, the paediatric nurse is committed to providing excellence in quality care that meets with the standards expected of the nursing profession. Commitment is about being loyal to the profession and the children to whom we care for. Commitment is also about dedication to continuing education, life-long learning, and becoming more skilled, socially conscious, ethical, politically competent, and caring.

Activity
Imagine you have just commenced working in a paediatric unit. What do you think you need to do to reflect a commitment to caring for children in the paediatric unit?

Comportment

Comportment is the way the health professional behaves as they go about caring for the patient. It is the way the health care professional presents themselves. Consider the nurse caring for the paediatric patient. They walk into the child's room. The parent is present. The nurse is well groomed, their uniform is clean and well pressed, their body language portrays confidence. They greet the child and the parent warmly and introduce themself. They go on to explain the plan of care for the shift as they go about doing safety checks. The nurse speaks to the parent in a respectful professional manner and communicates to the child at a level that the child understands. These attributes of dress, communication, behaviour, self-awareness, and accepting responsibility for one's own actions are all about comportment.

Activity
Reflect on someone whom you have the utmost respect for as a health care professional. What is about them? How do these factors equate to comportment? Is there something that you can take from this reflection that you can manifest in your own practice?

Creativity

Creativity as a health care professional in the caring context is about having the insight and ability to have a vision of seeing how things could be and going about making things better. I believe every person can be creative. Every health care professional can think about doing something in their practice that might make a difference for the patient. To do so may take courage, being resourceful, taking risks and learn something new if things do not work out as anticipated. It is about being resilient, flexible, and tenacious to have another go. Being creative is also about building on existing knowledge and finding new ways of doing things. As a nurse I have taken great pride in daring to be different by developing creative educational strategies and then sharing these with others. Two examples are the use of puppets with Pup-Ed™ (KRS Simulation) [4] and 'The Poop it Kit™' [5].

The Puppet Example: Pup-Ed™ (KRS Simulation)

In 2008 I began using puppets in the paediatric ward. I first started using cloth puppets that could be easily worn over my hand. The puppets were silent, they would whisper to me as I interacted with children. The rationale for this was so that the puppet was shy and vulnerable, hence promoting a human connection with the child. Additionally, I did not have a voice and the puppet could instead whisper what it wanted to say, and I would then channel that conversation. The puppet often had a condition that mirrored what the child had so in some ways could relate to the child. After doing this for several months, I decided to write down what I was doing and the reactions from children. Soon this would develop into what I would articulate as Pup-Ed™ (KRS simulation). This simulation technique, in essence, requires the puppets to be worn by a wearer who is an informed professional (for example the nurse). The professional then transforms the puppet into a little person with a history and story that becomes relevant to the child's experience. The puppet then becomes the platform for learning and teaching. The acronym stands for: P—puppet and professional preparation; U—understanding the learner; P—play in action to suspend disbelief; E—evaluation; D—debrief. The KRS component stands for knowledgeable, realistic, and spontaneous simulation. The knowledgeable implies that the wearer of the puppet has a deep understanding of the content being imparted through the puppet to the learner and appreciates different learning styles. Realistic suggests that the user creates a puppet experience which mimics a real situation. For example, in nursing, the professional wearing the puppet—(being the nurse), can draw upon episodes of patient care that a child may encounter. Spontaneous implies that the reaction of the puppet is unprompted. However, the puppet is directed by the professional who is in turn influenced by the learner response. Because scripts are not set, the reactions can be immediate in response to learners.

The Poop it Kit™

'The poop it kit™ is a resource designed for children and their caregivers to gain an understanding of bowel functioning and ways to promote healthy bowel habits. The contents of the kit included six books, a user guide, a board game, and a toilet wall poster.

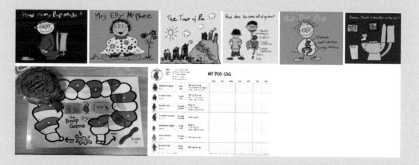

The resources focused on the anatomy and physiology of the intestinal system, prevention of constipation, diet to promote healthy bowel functioning, correct positioning on the toilet, ignoring the urge to go and holding on including fears about going to the toilet. Language used was designed to evoke laughter and enthusiasm. For this reason, words such as 'poop', 'bum', and 'fart' were included in the books and game. The images in the books were designed to be simple and easily relatable to the child. Gaps in the dialogue of the books were in place to allow the reader to include the child's name so that there was a sense that each book was personalized. At the conclusion of each book there were key points for the readers to raise with the child that could lead to further discussion.

Implementing Play through the Art of Caring

All the elements of caring previously discussed are centrals to play. So how do health care professionals bring play into their everyday practice? I believe nurses can provide a range of opportunities and experiences that foster different types of purposeful play to help children build understanding and reasoning.

So where does one start? The first might be to identify the literature that supports play as the 'work' of children. This includes acknowledging that play helps manage stress in a child's life [6] that it decreases anxiety, assists the child to adapt and cope with reality, and facilitates communication [7–9]. Further literature to consider includes the different stages of child development such as Jean Piaget [10] and Vygotsky's Zone of Proximal Development [11].

Understanding a child's stage of development can help health care professionals consider the type of play appropriate for the child. Studies undertaken by Parten

[12] revealed that children from 0–6 years participate in six different stages of social play which is determined by their stages of development. These include:

Unoccupied Play This is when the child observes, is not engaged in playing with others and makes sense of their world through manipulating materials. An example might be the child in hospital singing quietly to themselves or stroking a teddy.

Solitary Play This is when the child is engaged in their own play and is not interested in others. They explore freely developing motor and cognitive skills. An example might be the child in hospital playing with building blocks, Lego or colouring in.

Onlooker Play This is when the child observes others playing but does not engage or interact with the activity. During this stage the child is learning about social rules of play and relationships. An example might be the child in the hospital ward play area watching me interact with other children using puppets, or another child playing with blocks or a game.

Parallel Play This is when the child plays independently but alongside others. They may imitate the actions of others but do not engage in social interactions. An example might be the child in a play area of a hospital copying another child with blocks but not interacting with them.

Associative Play This is when the child is interested in others playing but does not engage in co-ordinating or organizing the play situation. An example might be the child in the hospital playroom sharing a play kitchen, playing dress-ups, or using the play equipment.

Co-Operative Play This occurs in later stage from 4 to 6 yrs. when the child is interested in both the activity and others playing and begins to establish shared rules for play. An example might be the child playing the game of 'The Poop it Kit™'. The child plays with other children learning the rules and how to win the game.

Smilansky's [13] identifies four different types of play linked to stages.

- Functional Play (1–2 yrs) where children explore their surroundings using their 5 senses.
- Constructive Play (2–3 yrs) where children build, assemble, and create using objects such as blocks, playdough, and craft items.
- Dramatic Play (3 +) where children engage in role play.
- Games with rules for children over 5.

Activity

Considering Smilansky's [13] different types of play and the stages, what items might you give:

The hospitalized 1–2-year-old to facilitate functional?
The 2–3-year-old in a health clinic to facilitate constructive play?
The 4-year-old in the day care centre to facilitate role play?
The 7-year-old in the hospital setting?

Understanding child development and the stages and categories of play are important because they have relevance to realistic expectations and the choice of toys, activities, and games that health care professionals can provide for children. However, to implement play from a health care professionals' perspective often requires a level of personal and professional reflection. The next section requires you to undertake some personal reflection.

Critical Reflection

To understand perspective about play requires one to reflect on their own beliefs and personal narrative including factors that enhanced play or hindered it. For some health care professionals, finding their inner child and being joyful in play may be effortless, especially if they have fond memories of play within their own family system. For others, this may not be the case and therefore being playful, scaffolding and directing children through different types of play may be challenging.

I reflect on what I believe enables or inhibits health care professionals from promoting, scaffolding, directing, and engaging in play with children. Three headings come to mind. These are:

1. the individual's belief system, knowledge, and skill set,
2. the context,
3. the child.

The Individual's Belief System, Knowledge, and Skill Set

An individual's belief, knowledge, and skill set pertaining to play is likely to be influenced by their own experiences as a child, the value of play within their family and cultural systems, their understanding of play, their personality, and their confidence. Influencing factors can also include their perception of what they believe their role is to play as a health care professional, what resources they have, and where play is situated in their current lives.

Activity

Take time to consider your own belief system, knowledge, and skill set about play. What shapes you in how you implement or not implement play around children.

*   What do you think are some of the barriers to play?*

The following is a list of tips that may be useful in your journey of implementing play as a health care professional.

Tips
- Take time to broaden your knowledge about play and its benefits.
- Consider the implications of play and stages of development.
- Reflect on your own childhood—find photos of yourself as a child and think back to what you loved to do.
- Give yourself permission to play in all its realms—imaginative and socio dramatic, constructive, and investigative, explorative, sensory (using the list above).
- Look for simple props—i.e. a hat, a pair of glasses, a wig and engage in role play.
- Find a space where you can let go of inhibitions—find your inner child.
- Be confident that engagement in play is important to the child and their caregiver.
- Look for 5-minute opportunities to engage in play.
- Make play a part of your busy day.
- Find simple resources and strategies—a piece of paper and pen, a balloon, a puppet, all can do wonders.
- Ask children what their favourite games are.
- Collaboratively create a story book with the child as the main character.
- Gather some paints, paper, and create—it doesn't matter if you think you are not an artist—just do it (you can even draw with your eyes closed).

The Context

The context includes the environment and the individuals within that setting.

The environment: It is an important consideration to promote and encourage play. It is not necessary to have an elaborate set-up with lots of toys, rather have a space that is aesthetically pleasing and encourages children to want to play. I have painted walls, ceilings, and doors in various health care settings with cartoon characters. The images were intended to send messages to children that this was their space. In considering the environment, I believe it is necessary to have tables, chairs, and beds at children's height. Simple resources such as books, balloons, paper, crayons, paints, boxes, blocks, and games are all useful items to promote play.

The individuals within the setting—attitudes:

The attitudes of individuals within the health care setting can influence others and their willingness to participate in play. It is realistic to state that nurses as health care professionals are busy, workloads can be heavy, and some would argue that there is little time for play. If some nurses believe that play is not in their role description, but rather the work of play therapists, then attitudes can impact on other individuals who understands the therapeutic and developmental benefits of play. The individual who wants to engage in play may be perceived as lazy because they are spending too much time with the child. Findings from a research study confirm this. In 2016 puppets were implemented in a regional paediatric setting in Queensland. The research examined nurses' experiences in using puppets over a 12-month period. The results revealed that whilst some nurses were happy to pick the puppets up, engage and play with children, others expressed that they lacked confidence in doing so or they were worried about other staff attitudes and believed if they played with the puppets they would be perceived as being lazy [4].

Tips to address attitudes
- Seek out like minded individuals in the unit who value play, and start brainstorming ideas.
- Look for ways to engage in play during all shifts.
- Find opportunities for dress-up days and make it an all-engaging opportunity.
- Present your ideas for play at staff meetings and seek out perceived challenges and ways to address them.
- Talk to peers and seek out like-minded individuals.
- When you see play being implemented in the ward, talk to those implementing it and seek out their ideas.
- Search for simple strategies and fun games that could be simply used in your facility.
- Make play a part of your everyday interaction.

The Child

Without doubt a strong factor influencing whether the health care professional will engage in play is the response of the child to the health care professional. It is important to remember that every child is different and how they respond to their situation in health care will be influenced by many factors including:

- The condition the child has.
- Medications.
- Anxiety.
- Pain.
- Other health-related conditions.
- Separation from family.
- Age.
- Language.
- Disability.

- Learning style.
- Confidence.
- Play ability.
- Other significant relationships.

Gaining an appreciation of the individual differences between children, having insight into what they may be going through in their health care journey will help position you in a space to engage and think about ways to implement play. Some simple strategies are listed below.

Tips to address the child
- Find out about the child—what is their name, condition, drugs, family situation.
- Look for ways to engage the child using age appropriate strategies.
- Consider pain relief if the child is uncomfortable.
- Respect privacy.
- Consider age-appropriate games.
- Seek out support from the family.

Caring for Yourself as You Engage in Play with the Hospitalized Child

Taking time to care for children and their families with the incorporation of play can be energy depleting both mentally and physically. It is important to recognize this and build some strategies for self-care. Consider the following:

- Do not take things personally if the child:
  - dismisses your offer of play
  - rejects your offer of resources for play,
- Remember if you engage in play not all your peers will place the same value on it as you do.
- Always consider the child's situation and their willingness to play—are they distressed, in pain, feeling nauseous, frightened or on pain relief medications?
- When feeling challenged about fostering play with the child when you have many competing work-place factors—remember the things that keep you motivated. Examples include:
  - A thank-you from an anxious mother.
  - A procedure that you have made less traumatic for the child through play.
  - The child that presents you with a thank-you drawing.
  - The difference you have made in a child's day.
- Be mindful also of your own journey and your experiences of play. There may be events in your role as a health care professional that triggers a negative feeling or on a positive side one of satisfaction. Above all, health care professionals are in a privileged position when caring for children and their families at a time when

they are most vulnerable. You can truly make a difference in caring for children in a developmentally sensitive approach and a central ingredient is the inclusion of play.

Conclusion

Caring for children in the role of a health care professional is a privilege. Caring encompasses compassion, competence, conscience, confidence, commitment, compartment, and creativity. Implementing play is part of caring. Every health care professional should consider play as part of the child's world and this should not cease for the child who is unwell, hospitalized or on a health care journey. As adults we may at times lose focus by being caught up with aspects that prevent us from encouraging play. Critical reflection in the context of personal life experiences and the courage to implement strategies to capture play is important.

References

1. Roach, M. S. (1984). *Caring: The human mode of being, implications for nursing*. Ottawa: The Canadian Hospital Association Press. ISBN 0-7727-3740-1.
2. Roach, M. S. (1992). The human act of caring: A blueprint for health professions.
3. Roach, M. S. (2002). Caring, the human mode of being: a blueprint for the health professions (2nd rev. ed.). Ottawa: Canadian Healthcare Association Press. Copy from Archives of Caring in Nursing, Christine E. Lynn College of Nursing, Florida Atlantic University, ARC-005 Sister M. Simone Roach Papers, 1958-2005, used by permission.
4. Reid-Searl, K., Quinney, L., Dwyer, T., Vieth, L., Nancarrow, L., & Walker, B. (2017). Puppetsin an acute paediatric unit: Nurse's experiences. *Collegian, 24*(5), 441–447. https://doi.org/10.1016/j.colegn.2016.09.005
5. Reid-Searl, K., Anderson, C., Crowley, K., Blunt, N., Cole, R., & Suraweera, D. (2021). A nursing innovation to promote healthy bowel functioning in children. *Collegian, 29*(2), 179–187.
6. Wong, D. L., Perry, S. E., Hockenberry, M. J., Lowdermilk, D. L., & Wilson, D. (2006). *Maternal child nursing care* (3rd ed.). Mosby Elsevier.
7. Ball, J., Bindler, R., Cowen, K., & Shaw, M. (2017). *Principles of pediatric nursing caring for children* (7th ed.). Pearson Education.
8. Caleffi, C., Rocha, P., Anders, J., Souza, A., Burciaga, V., & Serapião, L. (2016). Contribution of structured therapeutic play in a nursing care model for hospitalised children. *Revista Gaucha De Enfermagem, 37*(2), E58131.
9. He, H., Zhu, L., Chan, S., Liam, J., Li, H., Ko, S., et al. (2015). Therapeutic play intervention on children's perioperative anxiety, negative emotional manifestation and postoperative pain: A randomized controlled trial. *Journal of Advanced Nursing, 71*(5), 1032–1043. https://doi.org/10.1111/jan.12608
10. Piaget, J. (1976). Piaget's theory. In *Piaget and his school* (pp. 11–23). Springer.
11. Bruner, J. (1984). *Vygotsky's zone of proximal development: The hidden agenda*. New directions for child development.
12. Parten, M. B. (1932). Social participation among pre-school children. *The Journal of Abnormal and Social Psychology, 27*(3), 243–269.
13. Smilansky, S. (1968). *The effects of sociodramatic play on disadvantaged preschool children*. John Wiley & Sons.

Assessing the Sick, Injured, or Vulnerable Child

Belinda J. Dean, Judi A. Parson, and Karen Stagnitti

Objectives

At the end of this chapter, you will be able to:

- Consider the child within the family and health system to increase advocacy.
- List therapeutic play strategies which support the child to feel safe through orienting the child to the health setting environment.
- Identify at least three specific play assessments.
- Reflect on current practices and consider how therapeutic play assessment practices could be integrated.

Introduction

When a child needs access to health services, the first step is to assess the immediate health concerns for the child and triage accordingly. Once the child is considered physiologically stable, the clinician builds therapeutic rapport and communicates with the child and family in a developmentally sensitive manner. This commences at the first moment of interaction and the clinician is cognisant that this could be the child's very first presentation to a health setting. This experience could determine how the child will appraise future health care interactions and therefore has long-term implications. Often parents are asked questions about their child, but it is also

B. J. Dean (✉) · J. A. Parson · K. Stagnitti
School of Health and Social Development, Deakin University, Geelong, VIC, Australia
e-mail: belinda.dean@deakin.edu.au

© The Author(s), under exclusive license to Springer Nature
Switzerland AG 2022
J. A. Parson et al. (eds.), *Integrating Therapeutic Play Into Nursing and Allied Health Practice*, https://doi.org/10.1007/978-3-031-16938-0_4

important to listen to the voice of the child in the context of all interactions, including assessment and subsequent medical procedures or clinical treatments. The voice of the child includes play behaviours as well as verbal and nonverbal expression. This requires the clinician to have authentic, timely and strong observational and therapeutic skills to work with the child and family.

This chapter commences with acknowledging the highest priority when a child enters a health care setting—supporting life. Physical health is usually the foremost consideration for the child and authors agree it must take precedence; however, it should not be at the expense of psychological health and well-being. From the physical and psychological perspectives leads to an ever-widening systemic lens. The importance of interpersonal relationships is presented between the child, their family and health professionals to promote psychological safety. Following immediate considerations, child friendly and developmental sensitive aspects of assessment are discussed in the context of integrating therapeutic play strategies, including specific play assessments, which may be utilised in hospital and community health care services.

Immediate Treatment

When a child engages with the health system the child and their family may feel overwhelmed, stressed, and anxious, therefore the health professional can support the family by creating a relaxed stance and minimise potential stressors. When assessing the sick, injured, or vulnerable child, a chain of assessment events must take place to ensure their immediate health is prioritised. A child who is critically unwell must have their initial assessment needs met to ensure they return to a physiologically stable state. A general paediatric assessment, The Paediatric Assessment Triangle (PAT) is a simple diagnostic tool which assists to quickly assess the paediatric patients' current condition in an emergency [1]. Given the specific nature of assessing an infant, child, or adolescent, many generic adult scales or scoring systems are not suitable and typical ways of assessing an adult need to be adapted for paediatric populations [2]. Dieckmann et al. [1] stated that the development of PAT allows the practitioner to quickly understand the severity of the child's condition as well as determine the acuity of treatment and create a general impression to the multidisciplinary team. The main aim of the PAT is to determine how well or unwell the child is through assessing the child's appearance and vital signs. Once the child is determined to be physiologically stable and safe in the environment, then a more in-depth physical and neurological examination may be conducted.

Physical and Neurological Assessment

Many traditional measurements to assess children are non-distinct from adult assessment. These include, for example a head-to-toe physical assessment, including a neurological appraisal, in nursing or the conceptual model of human occupation in occupational therapy [3]. More recently, some assessments have been adapted to be paediatric specific [1, 2], however, more specific assessments require adaptations to be aligned with the paediatric population. Children may be difficult to assess as they may be distressed, frightened, or unwilling to participate when conducting a standard assessment screen. Additionally, their condition can deteriorate rapidly due to physiological immaturity and non-specific symptomology [1, 2]. Many traditional assessments remain crucial tools for assessment and measurement, particularly paediatric adaptions of instruments. This chapter argues that playful measures can be put in place which ensure the child feels comfortable, safe, and secure and therefore result in more accurate outcomes as the child is in a regulated state and not just willing, but keen to engage.

Pain Assessment and Experience

Witnessing children in pain is difficult and health care professionals are at risk of developing compassion fatigue. Being able to support the child to cope with pain can be rewarding. Assessing pain is the first step in working out a bespoke pain management plan. Pain assessments remain age dependent with different measures for infants, toddlers, school aged and adolescent patients [4]. Because pain is influenced by multiple factors it requires a systematic approach to assess, measure, and plan to cope with the pain [5]. The four features of pain experience include: (1) *nociception*, the physiological action that alerts the central nervous system to aversive stimuli; (2) *pain*, the sensory perception of the signal; (3) *suffering*, the emotional response to the painful episode, such as fear associated with a threat, and (4) *pain behaviour,* the actions associated with the response to pain [6]. The pain features may be used to target specific aspects for assessing the pain experience.

Pain scale assessments give the clinician a visual guide as to how the child assesses their own level of pain. Some examples of these include the Faces Pain Scale – Revised (FPS-R) and the Wong-Baker FACES pain rating scale where children point to a face that depicts their experience of pain [7]. For older children and adolescents, verbal numerical rating scales may be used where children rate their pain from 0 to 10 [4]. These scales are beneficial assessments as they can be used as comparative measures before and after a pain management intervention.

It is important to observe the child for signs of pain and compare this with usual pain behaviours at home or school. When approaching the child, a therapeutic stance is paramount to reduce any potential anxiety or fear associated with pain or other unknown factors. Is the child interacting with a family member, are they silent or sleeping, are they reading, hiding, or playing a game? What facial expressions are potential cues to observe when approaching the child.

Integrating Therapeutic Play into Clinical Assessments

Pharmacological and nonpharmacological approaches are tailored to the individual based on their physiological and subjective experience. Non-pharmacological approaches include therapeutic play interventions to support pain management to reduce the sensory perception of the pain through distraction or the emotional experience of suffering.

Some examples include using a puppet to demonstrate playful breathing techniques, incorporating music for guided imagery, use of digital or immersive virtual reality apps (see additional resources and Chap. 10), and consideration of sensory preferences as well as age-appropriate distraction techniques and comfort positioning and holding [4].

Assessing Neurobiology

Historically, the biomedical model considered the parts of the body separately as psychological and biological. This reductionist model is useful when assessing multiple pieces of physical health to distinguish critical information. A neurobiological assessment consists of examining the physical and mental state of the child or adolescent. The Glasgow Coma Scale (GCS) is an objective way to describe the levels of consciousness to assess children's responsiveness through eye-opening, motor, and verbal responses [8]. Neurological assessment includes shining a light into the child's eyes to check for pupil dilation, consciousness and arousal level, orientation to person, place and time, with age-appropriate modifications as well as a mental state exam observing the child's appearance and behaviours, mood, affect, speech, thought form and content, perception, insight and judgement, sensation and cognition as well as any further relevant psychosocial assessments [9].

Neurological assessment is used to assess the child's level of consciousness, movement and sensation, consciousness, and affect. Assessments view the child in how they present in the moment. Understanding neurosequential development is important when assessing the child in the context of their clinical situation against typical development. Neuroscientists have examined the critical periods of brain development in relation to early life trauma or disrupted attachment [10]. This is relevant to the health care setting because it also considers iatrogenic, procedural, treatment related medical trauma also known as Paediatric Medical Traumatic Stress (PMTS) (Christian-Brandt et al., 2019). The following Fig. 1 aligns the type of play associated with the critical periods of brain development as well as each of the psychosocial stages. This graphic has become a useful guide for clinicians to consider critical stages of development. What is important is that children who may have experienced early life trauma, or hospitalisation, or are currently unwell, may regress in their play to an early stage of development.

Having a deeper understanding of what has happened to the child in a specific developmental period may inform further assessments and what additional therapeutic support is required to ensure they continue to attain developmental

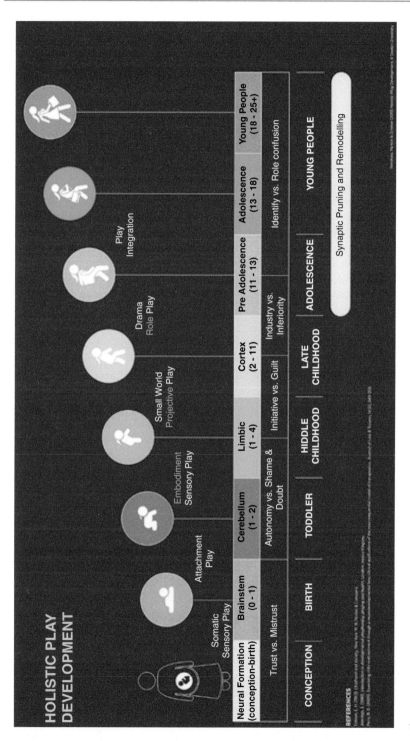

Fig. 1 Renshaw, Parson, and Zimmer (2019) Holistic play development. © Deakin University

milestones. There are a range of play-based assessments that can measure many areas of neurodevelopment including levels of play development. Section three presents many relevant assessments to support deeper understanding of a child's neurodevelopment, attachment, adverse experiences, and play ability.

Assessing Play

Assessing play in a clinical setting may seem an oxymoron because play is not associated with formality [11]. Play is a broad concept for many activities that a child engages in, such as catching a ball, dressing up for role play, or expressing through art and music. Play is a complex activity that appears deceptively simple [12]. Because play is complex, a play assessment of a child can provide rich information regarding how the child understands their world and how they function in it. Assessing play in a clinical setting is possible when the play assessment focusses on the unique attributes of play and the child's ability to self-initiate play [12]. The health care professional should consider developmentally, and culturally appropriate, play materials and their rationale for undertaking the play assessment. Pretend play (also called imaginative play or make-believe play) is essentially play [12]. All definitions of play include transcending reality and in pretend play a child is imposing meaning on what they are doing by attributing properties to objects (e.g. the teddy is naughty), referring to absent objects (e.g. it is raining), and using toys and objects as symbols in play (e.g. the box is a car), creating coherent stories, and purposefully planning what they wish to play.

Assessments of play that may be used within a some health care setting include: Pretend Play Enjoyment Developmental Checklist (PPE-DC) [13] which gives scoring indicating an age equivalent of play, enjoyment of play, and an emerging sense of self for children 12 months to 5 years; the Child-Initiated Pretend Play Assessment (ChIPPA) [14] which provides a norm score comparison for a child's quality of spontaneous play for children aged 3–7 years; or the Animated Movie Test (AMT) for children aged 8–15 years [15]. To carry out a play assessment in a clinical setting the environment needs to be a quiet room with few distractions. The child is invited to play and introduced to the play materials. In a play assessment, the examiner needs to create a feeling of safety for the child and this can be achieved by being aware of the physical space between the examiner and the child and sitting to the side of the child. The child may be anxious and so being further away is more comfortable for these children. The examiner uses a steady gentle tone, has an open body stance, and smiles with their eyes and mouth [16]. In these play assessments, the examiner is passive for most of the time and observing and scoring the child's play.

Application of Play Assessments in Health Settings

Utilising the play assessments such as the ChIPPA has been used to compare the quality and the quantity of pretend play ability of preschool-aged children who had experienced an acquired brain injured with their neurotypical peers (Thorne,

Stagnitti and [17]). Assessment of pretend play ability can inform clinical interventions rehabilitation and may be useful to ensure play development and enhance neurodevelopment. There are other types of developmentally sensitive assessments that may be standardised or non-standardised. These may focus on the child's strengths and difficulties, mental health concerns and provide insights into the child's current thoughts and feelings. The health care professional may also draw on assessment information provided by the family system. In part 3 of this text, a range of assessments have been integrated into clinical care. For example, Perrin (chapter 11) includes the Emotional safety framework – Psychosocial Risk Assessment in Paediatrics (PRAP); Sarah (Chap. 12) introduces the 6-Part Story Making (6PSM) and the BASIC Ph; Renshaw (Chap. 13) includes the Strengths and Difficulties Questionnaire (SDQ), Adverse Childhood Experiences (ACEs), Pediatric ACEs and Related Life Events Screener (PEARLS); and other creative arts techniques. Dean (Chap. 14) includes the Russ Affect in Play Scale.

The Child within the System

When meeting a child, for the first time consider what is already known about the child and their family. What assumptions could be made, e.g. age and stage of development, gender, race, and cultural heritage, presenting condition or family relationships? Purnell's model provides a useful graphic to identify the different cultures and issues that healthcare professionals need to be sensitive to [18]. The model is useful to appraise any potential cultural bias. Bronfenbrenner's bioecological systems theory is another useful model to conceptualise the physiological and psychological aspects of the child in the context of relational experiences and sociocultural factors [19, 20]. This model then situates the child within a broader health perspective that encompasses the child's system in a particular point in time. A considerate clinician "reads the room" when the child and family arrive as they assess the situation from a multilayer perspective.

Activity

Review the case example of Jessee (pseudonym) and reflect on the bioecological factors that may be impacting this scenario.

Jessee is a nine-year-old child that presents to your service. Jessee was triaged and you are now the assessing clinician. As you call for Jesse you note the child's appearance to be that of a Caucasian Australian, with red hair, who is exceptionally tall compared to their age group. You note that they are wearing a basketball jersey and basketball shorts with only one shoe. Jessee is accompanied by a tall adult of what appears to be an African descent who is helping Jessee. When observing the relationship between Jessee and the adult, you note that there seems to be some distance or discomfort between them, as if the adult does not feel comfortable to be so physically close to Jessee. As Jessee hops into the cubicle for assessment you consider if their foot or leg is injured. You also note Jessee's facial expressions indicate pain. The adult with Jessee seems deeply concerned. Jessee is silent and you need to ask clinical questions to find out more about Jessee, the presenting problem, and any other important bioecological factors within the family system.

Questions

What open-ended questions could you ask to find out more?
    Here's some to get you started:
    Clinician: "Nice to meet you Jessee, who have you brought in with you today?"
    Jessee explains that this is George, my coach.
    Clinician: "I can see by your clothes that you have basketball gear on......"
    Jessee: "yeah".
    Clinician: "I wonder if you might have hurt your foot playing basketball today, tell me what happened?"
    Jessee: "Can you tell 'em George".
    George: "Jessee went up to catch the ball and landed in a funny way".
    Clinician: "OK, thanks George, can you show me where it hurts, Jessee".

Reflections

- What do you already know about this child and adult?
- How much information do you have?
- What further information do you need?
- What are your assumptions towards this child/family/system?
- Did you note that no gender was mentioned for either Jessee or George, what assumptions did you make about this?
- What social and cultural considerations have you already factored in?
- Are you drawn towards wanting to address the physical condition before all else?

Building Rapport as an Interpersonal Assessment Skill

To build rapport with Jessee, the assessing nurse needs to create a sense of safety. To do this the health care professional appropriately responds to facial and body language cues, holds an open stance and uses culturally sound eye contact. These responses aim to support Jessee to be in a socially engaged state as opposed to a state of fear [21]. Jessee may be masking his true pain level, for example he may report a lower pain score to demonstrate his bravery, or he could be hypervigilant, and in shock which may impact on his ability to accurately assess his pain levels. The concept of neuroception is when the body signals if it is safe or in danger based on the perceived environment [22].
    The health care professional can then continue rapport building through therapeutic play-based ways of assessing, taking history, and considering environmental

and personal factors such as how child friendly the room is, how child friendly the clinician presents as being and how much external stimuli is happening as well as how Jesse is responding to this.

Activity Building Rapport: Helping the Child to Feel Safe

- Consider ways you could present yourself in your personal attire that would engage interest in children and/or adolescents. Consider wearing child friendly items of clothing (paediatric apron, colourful paediatric shoes, animal stethoscope, name badge with picture).
- Take time to be with the child to focus on rapport building. Consider the indigenous concept of yarning—storying that is cyclic and builds over time and turn taking. McCalman et al. [23] discuss the benefits of yarning as a community-driven, tested model that can support child and system outcomes.

Playful Approaches to Physical Assessment

Take time to explore the equipment which will be used in the assessment, for example show the child a thermometer, sphygmomanometer, stethoscope, or the pulse oximeter prior to using it and provide an explanation in a playful way. To do this the nurse may show the child how it will be used on a teddy, doll, or soft toy and then ask the child how the teddy, doll, or toy may feel about having the assessment. This communicates to the parent age sensitive ways to share information and normalise the experience together. If the child has the capacity, offer the child the pulse oximeter to put onto their own or their parent's finger. It is important to explain prior to putting it on the finger that the child may see a red light that shines through the skin and that the machine will make a beeping sound once it goes onto their finger. This can be supported with additional information about what the machine does and it detects how fast or slow the heart is beating. A stethoscope can also be used for the child to listen to their own heart (with assistance) to see if the beating is the same as the machine. Parents can be actively involved in this process depending on the age and developmental stage of the child. In terms of assent, a simple statement such as "we would like to put the finger probe on teddy now, does that sound ok teddy?" (ask the child if the Teddy says yes). Then "now we will put the finger probe on Mum, is that ok Mummy?" (Mummy says yes) and then "now we will put the finger probe on you, does that sound ok?" a head nod or yes is a form of assent. Be careful not to offer this as an option if the pulse oximeter needs to be put on the child at that very point in time or in an acute emergency. Instead, the child can give assent through providing an option. The practitioner can provide a statement such as "we are going to put the finger probe on now. Would you prefer it to go on your left hand or your right hand". When the child provides an indication of which hand they choose, this is their assent for the health care professional to continue. Options are always a great way of ensuring the child has choice which aligns with the UNCRC (see chapter 1) in the child having the right to say what should happen to them.

There are numerous types of assessment across health disciplines; however, what is most important is the approach and the health care professionals' curious and playful attitude towards the child. The playful stance can be applied to whatever assessment is being undertaken no matter the discipline. Vega and Hayes [24] speak of care, compassion, and communication as the core principles that create the art of nursing (see chapter 3). Being genuinely present and accepting the child's thoughts, feelings, and actions (within safe parameters) are humanistic ways of being with the child. Health care professionals should consider what they are bringing of themselves and consider how to effectively communicate through verbal and nonverbal means including listening actively to the wants, needs, and concerns of the child and respond to them directly in a child sensitive way. Bringing a playful stance along with professional expertise results in the art and science of nursing or other allied health care combining for the ultimate care experience. This way of being also supports the coming together of art and science within each profession within a multidisciplinary workforce [25]. Having a curious playful lens will assist with building rapport and helping the child to feel safe which will allow accurate biological measurements to be achieved. For example, an anxious child's pulse rate and respiratory rate may deviate from the resting pulse or respiratory rate. Keep in mind that some children find coming into hospital or a clinical setting to be exciting and may be curious or dysregulated depending on their previous experience and assumptions which may be real or unrealistic.

Activity: Setting Considerations

- How do you feel when you enter the room?
- What are your eyes first drawn to?
- Ask children what they notice first?
- Crouch down low and view things from the height of a child.
- Consider your own senses—what does it smell like, sound like, look like?
- Does anything look unusual, scary, worrying, or interesting?
- Can you see anything that is child friendly (pictures on the wall), are they at the eye level of the child or are they positioned for adults?
- Check the ceiling for when the child may lie on a bed.

Once you have thoroughly observed your environment, consider how you could make an eye spy game based on the examples below:
Situational eye spy game:

- How many doors are there? Include doors in and out as well as cupboards.
- What is the colour of the exit sign?
- Which direction takes you to bathroom or toilet?
- Is there a nurse call bell?
- How many lights can you count?
- What colour is the curtain?
- What can you hear?
- What can you smell? Does it smell nice or yucky?

Children may like to play hangman on a whiteboard, start of simple but then create some crazy spelling medical machinery, for example

- Sphygmomanometer.
- Stethoscope.
- Thermometer.
- Otoscope.

This can then open conversation about familiarisation with the medical equipment.

Conclusion

Assessing children is more complex than adapting an adult assessment for paediatric use. Therapeutic ways of working with children are required throughout the assessment process. The combining of the art and science of health ensures best practice outcomes for children requiring care. Children's immediate health concerns should be addressed as the highest priority to support life (ABCDE assessments). Once a child is viewed to be physically stable, neurological and pain assessments can be conducted in a play-based way as secondary assessments. Additionally, child play assessments can be used to assess development in diagnostic groups such as acquired brain injury and compared with neurotypical peers. The PPE-DC, ChIPPA, and AMT could be utilised further to evaluate treatment. Systemic factors such as neurobiological and play development should be considered and assessed.

Bronfenbrenner's systems theory can be integrated as a bioecological systems style of working with children, their families and the broader community encompassing the child. Purnell's model of cultural competence can ensure culturally sound practice.

The play-based therapeutic stance the clinician brings to the relationship will impact on the homeostatic state of the child and their functioning throughout the assessment period.

Additional Resources

- Your child's health and development – birth to 6 years: https://www.education. vic.gov.au/Documents/childhood/parents/health/chlchart6years.pdf
- The Royal Children's Hospital Melbourne – Clinical Guidelines (Nursing) Nursing assessment: https://www.rch.org.au/rchcpg/hospital_clinical_guideline_index/Nursing_assessment/#Admission%20Assessment
- The Royal Children's Hospital Melbourne – Clinical Guidelines (Nursing) Pain assessment: https://www.rch.org.au/rchcpg/hospital_clinical_guideline_index/Pain_Assessment_and_Measurement/

References

1. Dieckmann, R. A., Brownstein, D., & Gausche-Hill, M. (2010). The pediatric assessment triangle: A novel approach for the rapid evaluation of children. *Pediatric Emergency Care, 26*(4), 312–315. https://doi.org/10.1097/PEC.0b013e3181d6db37
2. Holt, K. (2009). Developing a triage tool for paediatric care: The use of existing triage systems is often inappropriate for children in emergency departments. Kerry Holt describes how a paediatric-specific triage tool was developed at her trust. *Emergency Nurse, 17*(3), 12.
3. Lee, S. W., Taylor, R., Kielhofner, G., & Fisher, G. (2008). Theory use in practice: A national survey of therapists who use the model of human occupation. *American Journal of Occupational Therapy, 62*(1), 106–117.
4. Wrona, S., & Czarnecki, M. L. (2021). Pediatric pain management an individualized, multimodal, and interprofessional approach is key for success. *American Nurse Journal, 16*(3), 6.
5. Liossi, C. (1999). Management of paediatric procedure-related cancer pain. *Pain Reviews, 6*(4), 279–302.
6. Fordyce, W. E. (1988). Pain and suffering: A reappraisal. *American Psychologist, 43*(4), 276–283.
7. Hockenberry, M. J., Rodgers, C. C., & Wilson, D. (2022). *Wong's essentials of pediatric nursing* (11th ed.). Elsevier.
8. Jain S, Iverson LM (2021 Jun 20). Glasgow coma scale. In *StatPearls [internet]*. StatPearls Publishing. 2022 Jan–. PMID: 30020670.
9. Realmuto, G., & Klimes-Dougan, B. (2012). Neurobiological assessment. In J. Kay & W. M. Klykylo (Eds.), *Clinical child psychiatry* (3rd ed.). John Wiley & Sons.
10. Perry, B. (2008). Child maltreatment: A neurodevelopmental perspective on the role of trauma and neglect in psychopathology. In T. Beauchaine & S. Hinshaw (Eds.), *Child and adolescent psychopathology* (pp. 93–129). John Wiley & Sons.
11. Stagnitti, K. (2022). Examining play in our pediatric clients: Formal assessments. In H. M. Miller Kuhaneck & S. L. Spitzer (Eds.), *Making play just right: Activity analysis, creativity, and playfulness in paediatric occupational therapy* (2nd ed.).
12. Stagnitti, K. (2004). Understanding play: The implications for play assessment. *Australian Occupational Therapy Journal, 53*, 3–12.
13. Stagnitti, K. (2017). *Pretend play enjoyment developmental checklist*. Learn to Play.
14. Stagnitti, K. (2019). *Child-initiated pretend play Assessment2*. Learn to Play.
15. Stagnitti, K. (2018). *Animated movie test*. Learn to Play.
16. Geller, S. M., & Porges, S. W. (2014). Therapeutic presence: Neurophysiological mechanisms mediating feeling safe in therapeutic relationships. *Journal of Psychotherapy Integration, 24*(3), 178–192. https://doi.org/10.1037/a0037511
17. Parson, J. A. (2021). Landscaping the therapeutic powers of play. In E. Prendiville & J. Parson (Eds.), *Clinical applications of the therapeutic powers of play: Case studies in child and adolescent psychotherapy*. Routledge.
18. Purnell, L. D., & Fenkl, E. A. (2019). *Handbook for culturally competent care*. Springer.
19. Bronfenbrenner, U. (2005). *Making human beings human: Bioecological perspectives on human development*. Sage Publications Ltd.
20. Sousa, R. C. R. D., Monteiro, E. M. L. M., Albuquerque, G. A., Paula, W. K. A. D., & Coriolano-Marinus, M. W. D. L. (2021). NURSING interventions to promote child development through Bronfenbrenner's bioecological theory. *Texto Contexto Enferm, 30*. https://doi.org/10.1590/1980-265X-TCE-2020-0685
21. Kestly, T. A. (2014). *The interpersonal neurobiology of play : Brain-building interventions for emotional Well-being*. W.W. Norton & Company. [2014].
22. Porges, S. (2021). Polyvagal theory: A biobehavioral journey to sociality. *Comprehensive. Psychoneuroendocrinology, 7*(100069). https://doi.org/10.1016/j.cpnec.2021.100069
23. McCalman, J., Bainbridge, R., James, Y. C., Bailie, R., Tsey, K., Matthews, V., Ungar, M., Askew, D., Fagan, R., Visser, H., Spurling, G., Percival, N., Blignault, I., & Doran, C. (2020).

Systems integration to promote the mental health of aboriginal and Torres Strait islander children: Protocol for a community-driven continuous quality improvement approach. *BMC Public Health, 20*(1), 1–12. https://doi.org/10.1186/s12889-020-09885-x

24. Vega, H., & Hayes, K. (2019). Blending the art and science of nursing. *Nursing, 49*(9), 62–63. https://doi.org/10.1097/01.NURSE.0000577752.54139.4e

25. Dean, B., & Parson, J. (2021). Integrating play-based approaches into nursing education: Teachers as playful academics. *Journal of Play in Adulthood, 3*(1), 71–86.

Attachment Theory in Paediatric Health Care

Natalie A. Hadiprodjo

Objectives

At the end of this chapter, you will be able to:

- Identify historical milestones in the development of attachment theory.
- Identify the different patterns of attachment.
- Reflect on the role of attachment in child and caregiver engagement in paediatric health care.
- Reflect on your own attachment history and how this may impact on the relationships you form with children and caregivers in the health care setting.

Introduction

This chapter explores how attachment theory may inform paediatric health care. The chapter provides a brief historical overview of attachment theory. It examines how a child's strategy of attachment may impact their response to medical care, and how parent strategies of attachment may impact parent engagement in the health care setting. It encourages paediatric health care professionals to work with caregivers to support attachment relationships between parents and children. The chapter includes activities to aid personal reflection and encourages the paediatric practitioner to consider their own attachment history, and how this may influence the relationships they form with the children and families in their care. An understanding of attachment theory can assist the health care professional to respond with compassion to stressed caregivers and children within the health care setting, and to tailor treatment to the needs of the child and family.

N. A. Hadiprodjo (✉)

School of Health and Social Development, Deakin University, Geelong, VIC, Australia

e-mail: natalie.hadiprodjo@deakin.edu.au

© The Author(s), under exclusive license to Springer Nature Switzerland AG 2022

J. A. Parson et al. (eds.), *Integrating Therapeutic Play Into Nursing and Allied Health Practice*, https://doi.org/10.1007/978-3-031-16938-0_5

A Brief History of Attachment Theory and Research

Reflective Activity
Think back to your own childhood. Who were the important attachment figures in your life? Who protected you as a child? Who did you go to for comfort? This may be a biological parent, grandparent, adoptive parent, foster carer, older sibling, or other important figure in your childhood.

Bowlby, Bombs, and Babies

Historically, attachment is a term used to describe the relationship between a caregiver and child, typically a mother and infant, but it also applies to intimate relationships across the lifespan. Attachment theory originated with the work of a British psychoanalyst and psychiatrist, John Bowlby, who defined attachment as a 'lasting psychological connectedness between human beings' [1, p. 194]. Bowlby is credited with seminal contributions to the field of attachment, fuelled by an interest in understanding the anxiety experienced by children separated from their primary caregiver. Bowlby examined the impact of children being sent away from their parents during WWII to escape the threat of bombings in London and concluded that separation from a parent was more threatening to a child's psychological wellbeing than bombs [2]. Bowlby's text on 'juvenile thieves' observed that extended separations from a mother during infancy may also contribute to criminal behaviour in adolescence [3]. Bowlby shone a light on the crucial role of attachment in a child's healthy psychological development. A central theme of Bowlby's work was the idea that a caregiver served as a secure base and haven, from which a child could explore the world and return to for comfort when the world proved frightening. Throughout his career Bowlby inspired and collaborated with a range of researchers and clinicians which shaped the evolution of attachment theory, from an early interest in security and separation, to a more nuanced understanding of individual differences in attachment relationships across the lifespan [4].

The Wire Mother Monkey

Reflective Activity
If you took a baby monkey, separated it from its biological mother, and placed it in a cage with a choice of two surrogate mothers—a soft cloth monkey or a wire monkey with a bottle of milk—who do you think the baby monkey would choose to spend more time with—the cloth monkey or the nursing wire monkey?
The above experiment was conducted in the 1950s by an American psychologist, Harry Harlow. Harlow conducted a range of what today would be considered unethical experiments terrifying small rhesus monkeys. While questionable, these experiments tested a common question in psychology at the time. Was the mother–infant bond primarily about food or comfort? A black and white documentary with stilted

dialect, gives insight into Harlow's research [5]. Harlow introduces a monkey called 'Baby 106' and narrates as Baby 106 goes to the nursing wire monkey for a quick suckle on the bottle. The infant monkey then returns to the cloth monkey where he clings to his surrogate mother as he rocks, squeaks, and sucks his thumb. In a tone of surprised discovery, Harlow explains that the monkey spends 17–18 hours a day with the cloth mother and less than 1 hour a day with the nursing wire monkey. A further experiment by Harlow involved a 'diabolical' robot, designed to frighten the infant monkey with its loud whizzing parts and sharp mechanical teeth. The infant monkey retreats to the cloth monkey, not the wire monkey, to sooth his fear. From this place of comfort, the emboldened monkey then turns to squark at the diabolical intruder. Similarly, if an infant monkey raised with the cloth and wire monkey, was placed in a strange room, they would nervously enter and cling to the floor. When the nursing wire monkey mother was introduced, the baby monkey took little notice and remained anxious. However, when the cloth monkey was introduced, the infant monkey quickly sought out and clung to the cloth monkey and then confidently went forth to explore the new room. The comfort provided by the cloth monkey enabled the infant monkey to then leave this secure base to explore the surrounds, capturing Bowlby's idea of a caregiver serving as a safe haven and a secure base from which an infant can explore the world.

A Two-Year-Old Goes to Hospital

Reflective Activity
A two-year-old child is left alone in a hospital for 8 days with no access to her parents. How do you think the child will respond? Will she scream and shout, or will she become silent and withdrawn?

If we view present-day medical care through the eyes of a child, these too are strange places filled with diabolical objects. Today we readily concede that the presence of a comforting caregiver is essential to easing a child's fear in a medical setting, but this was not always the case, as illustrated in another 1950s documentary that explored the plight of a child separated from her parents during a routine hospital admission. In post-WWII England it was commonplace for children to be admitted to hospital for long periods, without access to their parents due to fears of cross-infection and a belief that this was in the best interest of the child [6]. To highlight the emotional distress experienced by these children, James Robinson, a social worker in London, produced a film titled, *A Two-Year-Old Goes to Hospital* [7]. This film was unique in that it viewed this experience through the eyes of a two-year-old child Laura, following her separation from her mother for an eight-day admission. Laura responded to this separation as did Harlow's monkeys. Initially she was composed, then distressed, and then sunk into a state of despair and disconnect.

Robertson's film drew attention to the fact that 'young children need intimate contact with their parents, especially when they are ill. Fragmented care from changing nurses, however kind and friendly, is inadequate, causing upset and potentially unnecessary emotional damage' [8, p. 560]. Robertson and Bowlby became collaborators, working to identify the stages that a child progresses through when separated from their caregiver. Three stages were identified: protest, despair, and detachment [1]. While Robinson was not the only advocate calling for paediatric hospital reform, the visual and visceral nature of this film is credited with fuelling major reforms within paediatric health care. Robinson and Bowlby's work contributed to a parliamentary committee established by the British government to investigate the conditions in children's wards, which culminated in the Platt Report [9] that has influenced paediatric medical care across the developed world to the present day. The Platt Report outlined 55 recommendations including provisions for play and allowing parents to stay in hospital with their children during admissions [8].

The Strange Situation

In the 1970s the work of a psychologist Mary Ainsworth ushered in a new phase of attachment research. Until this point the emphasis in attachment studies had been on the negative effects of separation and the importance of a caregiver providing comfort and safety for healthy psychological development. This next phase of attachment research explored the idea that attachment relationships varied between infant–caregiver dyads. With Ainsworth's research came the realisation that there was not just one type of attachment, but multiple patterns or ways of being in relationship. Ainsworth's most renown experiment is the Strange Situation Procedure [10]. In this laboratory study, researchers observed infants between the ages of 12 and 18 months and their response to being placed in strange room with toys, initially with their mother. The study then follows a series of steps where a stranger enters the room, the mother leaves, the child remains with the stranger, the mother returns, the stranger leaves, the mother leaves, the child is left alone, and finally the mother returns [10]. Based on the parent's interaction with their child, and the reactions observed in the infants during the Strange Situation, Ainsworth identified three broad patterns of attachment labelled Type A, Type B, and Type C. Children coded as Type B displayed secure attachment behaviours. Children who displayed anxious attachment behaviours, showed two different and distinct patterns of attachment behaviour, labelled Type A and Type C. Within the attachment literature a Type A attachment may also be referred to as insecure avoidant or dismissive and Type C as insecure ambivalent, resistant, or preoccupied. Within this chapter the original Type A, B, and C classifications will be used to avoid the negative connotations that can come with the latter labels.

Type B Patterns

A balanced and secure attachment was labelled Type B. These children typically had parents who were sensitive, available, and responsive to their child's distress. Children who displayed Type B attachment behaviours during the Strange Situation showed distress when their mother left the room but were readily comforted on her return [10]. Children with a Type B strategy of attachment typically have caregivers who can help a child make cognitive and affective meaning of their experience [11]. These children learn that when they show distress, they can rely on their caregiver to respond, provide comfort, and help regulate their arousal. For these children they develop the idea that feelings can be shared, and that other people can be relied on to provide protection and comfort when needed [11].

Type A Patterns

One type of anxious attachment pattern was labelled Type A. These children had parents who were predicable but less sensitive and responsive to their distress within the Strange Situation. Children who displayed Type A attachment behaviours did not display distress when their mother left the room, nor did they seek comfort on her return [10]. Subsequent studies have shown that children who show Type A attachment behaviours do experience internal physiological distress, although this may not be visible [12]. These children have unconsciously learnt that outward displays of distress do not elicit a comforting response from their caregiver and may result in a caregiver pulling away or becoming distressed themselves [11]. For these children, they learn that they will garner a more favourable response from their caregiver if they inhibit their own distress [10]. Thus, infants with a Type A strategy show a preference for cognition and rules (for example, if I do this, then this happens) and a tendency to inhibit their affect, especially negative affect [11].

Type C Patterns

A further type of anxious attachment was labelled Type C. These children typically had parents who were inconsistent in their responsiveness, who were sensitive one moment and withdrawn or preoccupied the next. Children who displayed Type C attachment behaviours showed an opposite pattern of behaviour from those children categorised as Type A within the Strange Situation. These children showed visible, exaggerated distress when their parent left the room and were not easily comforted on her return [10]. These children had unconsciously learnt that outward displays of exaggerated distress were useful in maintaining a consistent and attentive response from a caregiver who may otherwise be distracted or inconsistent. Children with a Type C strategy show a preference for the expression of negative affect, and a tendency to disregard how they think and act on how they feel [11].

Contemporary Models of Attachment

Bowlby and Ainsworth's ideas informed the first theory of attachment, the Bowlby-Ainsworth Theory of Attachment. Two contemporary models of attachment have subsequently built on this theory and the A, B, and C classifications—the ABCD Model and the Dynamic Maturational Model of Attachment and Adaptation (DMM).

ABCD Model

In addition to the three styles of attachment identified by Ainsworth, researchers Hesse and Main [13] identified a group of infants who did not fit the A, B, C categories of attachment. These infants demonstrated bizarre behaviours during the Strange Situation and appeared conflicted, disoriented, or fearful [14]. These children were categorised as displaying a disorganised pattern of attachment, labelled Type D [15]. This model is thus referred to as the ABCD model of attachment. The term disorganised attachment has become widely used by clinicians and in popular culture, however, it is important to note that this term is often used outside of its intended purpose. Disorganised attachment is a research-based term specific to the Strange Situation [16] and should not be used for children above 20 months of age [14]. Children older than 20 months tend to develop more sophisticated and organised strategies of attachment (e.g. Type A or Type C). A further misconception is that a disorganised attachment is a certain indicator of childhood maltreatment. While a disorganised attachment coding within the Strange Situation is more common among children who have been maltreated, not all maltreated children demonstrate a disorganised attachment within the Strange Situation [16].

The Dynamic Maturational Model of Attachment and Adaptation

The DMM was developed by Patricia Crittenden. As in the name, this model focuses on the *dynamic*, *maturational*, and *adaptive* nature of attachment. All strategies of attachment are considered *adaptive* solutions to the difficulties individuals may face [4]. Through this lens, Type A, B, and C are protective strategies that help a child remain close to their caregivers. Within this model all strategies of attachment are considered adaptive to the context, with some strategies being organised around greater danger than others. However, strategies that are adaptive in dangerous environments may be less adaptive in a safe environment [17]. Crittenden emphasises that it is the strategy that is labelled and not the person. Attachment is not a trait that defines the whole person but indicates how an individual responds under stress [18].

Attachment strategies are also *dynamic* and can change across the lifespan, with more complex strategies becoming available as children develop into adulthood, thus the model is *maturational*. It is also possible to have more than one strategy of attachment and a child may have different strategies with different caregivers. Moreover, healthy relationships in adulthood have the capacity to reorganise and aid in the development of new strategies of attachment, so that an individual may become what is called 'earned secure' [17]. In the DMM there is no Disorganised or Type D category of attachment, but a more graduated and nuanced distinction in the Type A, B, and C strategies. The DMM is represented as a wheel or pie chart with a total of 12 sub-categories [17].

Type B is further sub-classified as:

- B1–2 Reserved.
- B3 Comfortable.
- B4–5 Reactive.

Type A is further sub-classified:

- A1–2 Inhibited/Socially Facile.
- A3–4 Compulsive Caregiving/Compliant.
- A5–6 Compulsively Promiscuous/Self-Reliant.
- A7–8 Delusion Idealisation/Externally Assembled Self.

Type C is further sub-classified:

- C1–2 Threatening/Disarming.
- C3–4 Aggressive/Feigned Helplessness.
- C5–6 Punitive/Seductive.
- C7–8 Menacing/Paranoid.

The final classification is AC Psychopathy. Within the model normative strategies include all Type B classifications, as well as A1–2, and C1–2 categories. While individuals utilising an A1–2 or C1–2 strategy may not be classified as secure, individuals who adopt these strategies are at less risk for psychopathology. The remaining strategies become increasingly complex as an individual develops, with the highest numbered strategies only becoming available in adulthood. These higher numbered strategies form in response to increasing danger and are associated with an increased risk for psychopathology [17].

The Application of Attachment Theory to Paediatric Health Care

Attachment strategies are activated during times of stress. Illness, injury, and medical intervention may activate attachment behaviours, much like the Strange Situation study. Attachment theory provides a framework for understanding the underlying reason for behaviours displayed by children and caregivers within the medical setting in response to stress. This understanding may assist the health care professional to act with greater compassion and may also inform how health care is adapted to the individual needs of the patient [19]. Attachment theory can also provide health care professionals with insight into their own responses to the children and families in their care. The following section will explore how an attachment lens may be applied to the health care professional, the child, and the caregiver.

Understanding the Health Care Professional

Reflective Activity
What are your motives for becoming a paediatric health care professional. What inspires you to work with children? Does this interest stem from your own childhood experiences?

The Adult Attachment Interview (AAI) is one measure that can be used to assess attachment in adulthood [17]. The AAI is a semi-structured interview that asks the interviewee to reflect on their childhood experiences. The interview is then transcribed and coded by a trained coder. It may be coded using the ABCD or DMM model. While the interview is coded as a whole, one question is especially relevant to health, where the interviewee is asked to reflect on what happened when they were ill or physically injured as a child. An individual operating from a Type B (balanced secure) strategy may share examples of how they sought help from a caregiver, who in turn provided both comfort and protection. Alternatively, an individual utilising a Type A strategy may instead focus on their own self-reliance and capacity to deal with the problem without the help of an adult, or describe a caregiver who discouraged the expression of emotional distress. They may also minimise childhood experiences of illness or injury and prioritise their caregiver's perspective and fail to acknowledge how painful or frightening this was for them as a child. In instances where injury was caused by a caregiver through abuse, the interviewee may seek to justify the caregiver's behaviour. Alternatively, an individual utilising a Type C strategy may prioritise their own perspective and may report revelling in their caregiver's attention when they were injured or unwell and may have even exaggerated their distress as a way of securing attention and comfort from their caregiver.

While health care professionals may draw on any of the strategies of attachment discussed, individuals drawn to the helping professions may have a great tendency to adopt a Type A3 (compulsive caregiving) strategy of attachment according to the DMM. Crittenden and Landini [17] observe that adults with a Type A3 strategy feel most comfortable when caring for others. Individuals with a Type A3 strategy may have taken on a caregiving role as a child, where they were required to care for and comfort a vulnerable caregiver, which theoretically leads to the tendency to take on caregiving roles in adulthood. Individuals with a Type A3 strategy tend to dismiss their own needs and focus on the needs of others and readily comply with rules and regulations. While these qualities may make for wonderful health care professionals in many ways, they may also lead to a tendency to cut off from one's own emotion and lead to a greater propensity for burnout and compassion fatigue. Studies have shown that health professionals utilising a secure attachment strategy are less prone to burnout and report greater job satisfaction [20].

One of the most hopeful features of attachment theory is the dynamic nature of attachment. All adults can develop additional more secure strategies of attachment. The defining feature of a secure attachment is not whether you have had difficult experiences as a child, but how you reflect, integrate, and tell your story. An individual with a secure attachment can tell a coherent story about their childhood and how these experiences have shaped them as an adult and a professional. They can take on numerous complex perspectives without avoiding the difficult parts of their story (Type A) or becoming overwhelmed by their own feelings (Type C) [17]. Health care professionals may benefit from taking time to reflect on their own childhood attachment experiences and in some instances, it may be beneficial to seek out a counsellor or therapist to help integrate these experiences.

Understanding the Child

The A, B, and C patterns or strategies of attachment can also aid in understanding the different behaviours children may display in the health care setting.

Type B Patterns

Children who display Type B (secure) attachment behaviours typically have caregivers who have been consistently responsive and attentive. These children experience low attachment anxiety and are more likely to see adults, including health care professionals, as sources of help. These children will be better equipped to deal with the stress of medical intervention and will be readily soothed and comforted by the presence of their caregiver. It is conjectured that these children will be able to accurately communicate their symptoms and level of discomfort while receiving medical care. As Crittenden [11] observes, these children tend to be open in their communication and able to express both positive and difficult feelings.

Type A Patterns

Children who display Type A attachment behaviours experience high attachment anxiety and a tendency to inhibit distress, to meet their attachment needs. In a medical setting, these children may seem overly calm or brave. These children may be less likely to view caregivers or health care professionals as a source of help or comfort and may present as overly self-reliant or pseudo-mature. These children are typically over-sensitive to the needs of their caregiver and may avoid expressing feelings that they perceive may upset their caregiver [11]. Therefore, these children may not show negative affect, cry, demand attention or report their pain or discomfort accurately. These children may show 'false positive affect' and appear smiley and happy on the surface, despite experiencing distress, pain, or discomfort [11]. These children will be easy to care for and highly compliant with medical procedures and may be perceived as the ideal patient and praised for their bravery. The risk for the health care professional is to assume that these children are coping well, when in fact, under the surface they may be experiencing significant distress.

Children utilising a Type A strategy of attachment will have a tendency towards cognition, logical reasoning and following the rules [11]. They will be eager to do the right thing when it comes to health care and medical procedures and will cognitively grasp the reasons for their medical intervention and what needs to happen and why. These children may benefit from being provided with choice, where possible, to enhance their feeling of independence [21]. These children will need permission and support to express their feelings, especially negative feelings. The use of metaphor, narrative, or symbolism through play could be used to engage these children as this provides a child with an avenue where they can express their inner world without the need to speak directly about themselves or their feelings. A child utilising a Type A strategy may find it easier to express their feelings through the character of a puppet or toy. Play provides a symbolic distance that allows children to explore difficult content without becoming overwhelmed or fearing that they will overwhelm others.

Type C Patterns

Children who display Type C attachment behaviours experience high attachment anxiety and a tendency to exaggerate distress, to meet their attachment needs. These children give more weight to feelings than cognition [11]. They may also keep a close eye on their caregivers and are vigilant to the outside world and may cling to caregivers and health care professionals. These children may report numerous symptoms, may be difficult to comfort, and may protest medical procedures. Therefore, they may be perceived as difficult to care for. While these children may be talkative, they may lack clarity and adults may struggle to understand what it is the child needs or wants. As Crittenden observes, language functions to keep others involved, rather than to clearly communicate a need [11]. These children will readily express their feelings and will need a greater level of emotional containment along with routine and predictability. Caregivers may need to be supported to respond to their child's distress in a calm and consistent manner [21]. Rather than support to express their feelings, these children will need help to see the connection between events and outcomes [11]. In the health care setting, these children may benefit from understanding the connection between their medical treatment and health outcomes.

Understanding the Caregiver

Finally, an attachment lens can be used to understand the caregiver.

Type B Patterns

Caregivers who operate from a Type B strategy of attachment will be in the best position to provide their child with a positive relationship that will strengthen the child's ability to cope with illness or injury. These parents will be able to hold their child's distress without becoming dysregulated themselves and will be able to make use of their own personal supports to effectively manage their own distress.

Type A Patterns

A caregiver operating from Type A strategy of attachment may approach their child's care in an intellectual fashion. They may seek out literature and be well versed in their child's condition, but this may also serve the purpose of shielding them from their child's distress or their own. These caregivers will be able to provide a coherent account of their child's medical history, but this may be presented in a matter-of-fact manner, with a tendency to minimise the difficulties experienced. These caregivers may be more rigid in their coping mechanisms and suppress negative emotion such as anger and fear. Caregivers with a Type A strategy may not be perceived by health care staff as problematic but may be considered controlling or avoidant [22]. These caregivers may benefit from being provided with choice and control where possible and an understanding of what is happening and why, along with clear and concrete instructions on what they can do to assist and comfort their child. These parents may need assistance in connecting with and responding to their child's fears and worries.

Type C Patterns

Caregivers operating from a Type C strategy may approach their child's care in a more emotive fashion. They may demand a lot of attention from medical staff and be overwhelmed by their own emotional needs and may catastrophise regarding their child's care. These parents may be less able to provide a coherent medical history and may provide a fragmented account that is difficult to follow. These parents may express strong emotions such as anger and aggression. This in turn may result in the health care worker feeling a desire to either rescue or pull away [22]. These caregivers may benefit from support groups, parent education, or counselling to help them manage their own emotions, along with regular times when they can meet with the treating team for support.

Further Considerations

Attachment and Medical Trauma

As evident in Laura's admission to hospital in the 1950s, parents play a vital role in providing comfort to children in the medical setting. A key role of the paediatric health care professional is to support parents to be a secure base and safe haven for their child. Engaging parents in the medical setting is a key means of guarding against medical trauma. Approximately 30% of children requiring medical care will develop symptoms of post-traumatic stress [23]. Frequent separation from caregivers for medical intervention has been identified as a risk factor for post-traumatic stress [24]. Medical trauma is defined by the presence of two features—overwhelming fear and a sense that you cannot escape [25]. In instances where a parent is involved in holding a child down for a medical procedure, studies have shown that these children present with more dissociative symptoms [26]. Dissociation is linked to the immobilisation freeze response and a greater propensity for developing PTSD [25]. If parents are to be involved in their child's medical care, where possible, this should be non-intrusive, with a focus on comforting the child and not assisting in the child's restraint.

It is also possible that chronic childhood illness may impact on the quality of an attachment relationship between a child and parent, especially where a child experiences long or frequent hospitalisations [27]. In instances where a child has a chronic illness, this may lead to lower levels of parental responsiveness and emotional warmth, and higher levels of control [27], like the features of a Type A pattern of attachment. It could also be hypothesised that a Type A strategy of attachment may be an adaptive means of coping with chronic illness for a child, given that this may require a child to cut off from uncomfortable feelings and endure medical procedures without the presence of a comforting adult. Further research is needed to ascertain the impact of medical care on attachment. However, in instances where medical treatment has adversely impacted on the attachment relationship between a caregiver and child, family interventions such as filial therapy may be helpful to repair and enhance the attachment relationship [28].

Attachment and Health Outcomes

While childhood medical intervention may impact on attachment security, attachment security may also play a role in health outcomes. Attachment relationships impact on the physiology of the stress response system. A child with a secure attachment can rely on their caregiver to help them regulate their physiological stress. A child with an insecure attachment is less able to rely on their caregiver to help them regulate their arousal and may therefore experience chronic physiological stress, that may in turn lead to an increased risk of future illness [29]. It is well established that adverse childhood experiences are associated with an increased risk for poor health outcomes in adulthood [30]. Insecure attachment is linked to more frequent ill-health and somatic complaints [21]. It is also possible that the different strategies of insecure attachment may be linked to a greater risk for specific health issues. For example, Baim and Morrison [31] observe that individuals who adopt a Type A strategy of attachment and suppress negative affect, may instead find these feelings somatically expressed through illness and depression. Alternatively, individuals who adopt a Type C strategy may be more at risk of engaging in dangerous behaviours to attract the attention of distracted caregivers, such as self-harm or substance abuse [31].

When Caregivers Harm

In some instances, children may present with illness or injury that has resulted from harm caused by their caregiver. In these cases, the caregivers themselves are the source of danger and these families will need to be provided with specialised intervention and referred to child protection services. It is not always easy for health care professionals to spot these highly vulnerable at-risk children and families. As discussed, children can become apt at presenting what they think others wish to see. Health care professionals should observe a child's behaviour and be on the lookout for incongruencies. If a child is inordinately happy following a terrifying experience resulting in significant injury, this may indicate that further investigation is warranted.

While an extreme illustration, the murder of eight-year-old Victoria Climbié in the UK serves as a warning for health care professionals. Despite several admissions to hospital during her abuse with numerous injuries that were suspected as non-accidental, Victoria was discharged to her abusive caregivers. While subsequent investigation highlighted numerous system flaws, this case has also been identified as an example of how a child's strategy of attachment may be misunderstood by health care professionals [32]. Victoria was perceived to be a friendly, happy child with a smile that lit the room. A hospital nurse observed that she would twirl up and down the ward. Following her death, the pathologist reported numerous injuries, the worst case of child abuse he had witnessed [33]. It is theorised that Victoria was utilising a compulsive Type A self-protective strategy of attachment according to the DMM [32]. Her smile was in fact a false positive affect that aimed to please others and hide her true pain and distress. This behaviour, while designed to shut down and deflect abuse by her caregivers, also had the effect of shutting down a protective response from the many professionals she encountered [32]. An understanding of attachment theory may aid the health care professional in not only understanding and adapting health care to the individual needs of children and caregivers within the health care setting—it may also equip practitioners to better detect children at risk.

Chapter Summary

This chapter explored how attachment theory may inform paediatric health care. The chapter provided an overview of the development of attachment theory from Bowlby to the present day and the different patterns of secure and insecure attachment. An attachment lens was applied to the child, caregiver, and health care professional. Health care happens in relationship and an understanding of attachment theory may aid in tailoring treatment to the individual and responding with compassion to stressed caregivers and children within the health care setting. A key role of the paediatric health care professional is to promote and protect healthy attachment between children and their caregivers, which in turn may guard against medical trauma and lead to enhanced health outcomes.

Reflective Questions and Activities

- Some of the content in this chapter is challenging and may touch on your own lived experience. You may wish to take some time to engage in a self-care activity or journal a response to this chapter. As noted, personal counselling or therapy can be helpful for the practitioner who wishes to gain greater insight into their own childhood and how this has shaped them as an adult and professional.

- How might an understanding of attachment theory inform your work with children and families in the future?

Additional Resources

- The Family Relations Institute https://familyrelationsinstitute.org/
- The National Child Traumatic Stress Network (NCTSN) www.NCTSNet.org

References

1. Bowlby, J. (1969). *Attachment. Attachment and loss: Vol 1. Attachment*. Basic Books.
2. Bowlby, J. (1951). *Maternal care and mental health. Monograph series, 2*. World Health Organisation.
3. Bowlby, J. (1944). Forty-four juvenile thieves: Their characters and home-life (II). *International Journal of Psycho-Analysis, 25*, 107–128.
4. Crittenden, P. M. (2017). Gifts from Mary Ainsworth and John Bowlby. *Clinical Child Psychology and Psychiatry, 22*(3), 436–422. https://doi.org/10.1177/1359104517716214
5. Baker, M. (2010, December 17). *Harlow's studies on dependency in monkeys* [video file]. YouTube. https://youtu.be/OrNBEhzjg8I
6. Alsop-Shields, L., & Mohay, H. (2001). John Bowlby and James Robertson: Theorists, scientists and crusaders for improvements in the care of children in hospital. *Journal of Advanced Nursing, 35*(1), 50–58.
7. Concord Media. (2014, July 1). *A two year old goes to hospital (Robertson films)* [video file]. YouTube. https://youtu.be/s14Q-_Bxc_U
8. Robertson, J., & McGilly, K. (2009). Comments on "Changing attitudes towards the care of children in hospital: a new assessment of the influence of the work of Bowlby and Robertson in the UK, 1940-1970" by Fank C. L van der Horst and Rene van der Veer (Attachment & Human Development Vol 11, No 2, March 2009, 119–142). *Attachment & Human Development, 11*(6), 557–561.
9. Minsitry of Health. (1959). *The welfare of children in hospital, Platt report*. Her Majesty's Stationery Office.
10. Ainsworth, M. D. S., Blehar, M. C., Waters, E., & Wall, S. N. (1978). *Patterns of attachment: A psychological study of the strange situation*. Psychology Press.
11. Crittenden, P. M. (2005). *Attachment and early intervention [keynote address]*. German Association of Infant Mental Health (GAIMH). Hamberg.
12. Holmes, J. (2009). *Exploring in security: Towards and attachment-informed psychoanalytic psychotherapy*. Routledge.
13. Hesse, E., & Main, M. (2000). Disorganized infant, child, and adult attachment: Collapse in behavioral and attentional strategies. *Journal of the American Psychoanalytic Association, 48*(4), 1097–1127. https://doi.org/10.1177/00030651000480041101
14. Main, M., & Solomon, J. (1990). Procedure for identifying infants as disorganized/disoriented during the Ainsworth strange situation. In M. T. Greenberg, D. Cicchetti, & E. M. Cummings (Eds.), *Attachment in the preschool years* (pp. 121–160). University of Chicago Press.
15. Main, M., & Solomon, J. (1986). Discovery of a new, insecure-disorganized/disoriented during the Ainsworth strange situation. In M. Yogman & T. B. Brazelton (Eds.), *Affect development in infancy* (pp. 95–124). Ablex.
16. Granqvist, P., Sroufe, L. A., Dozier, M., Hesse, E., Steele, M., van Ijzendoorn, M., Solomon, J., Schuengel, C., Fearon, P., Bakermans-Kranenburg, M., Steele, H., Cassidy, J., Carlson, E., Madigan, S., Jacobvitz, D., Foster, S., Behrens, K., Rifkin-Graboi, A., Gribneau, N., Spangler,

G., et al. (2017). Disorganized attachment in infancy: A review of the phenomenon and its implications for clinicians and policy-makers. *Attachment & Human Development, 19*(6), 534–558. https://doi.org/10.1080/14616734.2017.1354040

17. Crittenden, P. M., & Landini, A. (2011). *Assessing adult attachment: A dynamic-maturational approach to discourse analysis.* WW Norton & Company.
18. Chimera, C. (2010). An interview with pat Crittenden. *Context, 110,* 12–15.
19. Hunter, J., & Maunder, R. (2016a). Introduction. In J. Hunter & R. Maunder (Eds.), *Improving patient treatment with attachment theory: A guide for primary care practitioners and specialists* (pp. 3–7). Springer.
20. West, A. L. (2015). Associations among attachment style, burnout, and compassion fatigue in health and human service workers: A systematic review. *Journal of Human Behavior in the Social Environment, 25*(6), 571–590.
21. Feeney, J. A. (2000). Implications of attachment style for patterns of health and illness. *Child: Care, Health and Development, 26*(4), 277–288.
22. Hunter, J., & Maunder, R. (2016b). Advanced concepts in attachment theory and their application to health care. In J. Hunter & R. Maunder (Eds.), *Improving patient treatment with attachment theory: A guide for primary care practitioners and specialists* (pp. 27–37). Springer.
23. Forgey, M., & Bursch, B. (2013). Assessment and management of paediatric iatrogenic medical trauma. *Current Psychiatry Reports, 15*(2), 1–9.
24. National Child Traumatic Stress Network. (2014). *Pediatric medical traumatic stress. A comprehensive guide for health care providers.* Retrieved October 21, 2021, from https://www.nctsn.org/resources/pediatric-medical-traumatic-stress-toolkit-health-care-providers
25. Porges, S., & Daniel, S. (2017). Play and the dynamics of treating pediatric medical trauma. Insights from polyvagal theory. In S. Daniel & Trevarten (Eds.), *Rhythms of relating in children's therapies: Connecting creatively with vulnerable children.* Jessica Kingsley Publishers.
26. Disseth, T. H. (2005). Dissociation in children and adolescents as reaction to trauma - an overview of conceptual issues and neurobiological factors. *Nordic Journal of Psychiatry, 59*(2), 79–91.
27. Pinquart, M. (2013). Do the parent-child relationship and parenting behaviors differ between families with a child with and without chronic illness? A meta-analysis. *Journal of Pediatric Psychology, 38*(7), 708–721.
28. VanFleet, R. (2017). Family-oriented treatment of childhood chronic medical illness. The power of play in filial therapy. In L. C. Rubin (Ed.), *Handbook of medical play therapy and child life: Interventions in clinical and medical settings.* Tylor & Francis Group.
29. Maunder, R. G., Lancee, W. J., Nolan, R. P., Hunter, J. J., & Tannenbaum, D. W. (2006). The relationship of attachment insecurity to subjective stress and autonomic function during standardized acute stress in healthy adults. *Journal of psychosomatic research, 60*(3), 283–290. https://doi.org/10.1016/j.jpsychores.2005.08.013.
30. Felitti, V. J., Anda, R. F., Nordenberg, D., Williamson, D. F., Spitz, A. M., Edwards, V., Koss, M. P., & Marks, J. S. (1998). Relationship of childhood abuse and household dysfunction to many of the leading causes of death in adults: The adverse childhood experiences (ACE) study. *American Journal of Preventive Medicine, 14*(4), 245–258. https://doi.org/10.1016/S0749-3797(98)00017-8
31. Baim, C., Morrison, T., & Rothwell, B. (Collaborator). (2011). Attachment-based practice with adults: Understanding strategies and promoting positive change: A new practice model and interactive resource for assessment, intervention and supervision. Pavilion Publishing (Brighton).
32. Grey, B., & Gunson, J. (2019). Invisible children? How attachment theory and evidence-based procedures can bring to light the hidden experience of children at risk from their parents. In W. Bunston & S. Jones (Eds.), *Supporting vulnerable babies and young children: Interventions for working with trauma, mental health, illness and other complex challenges* (pp. 191–207). Jessica Kingsley Publisher.
33. Laming, L. (2003). *The Victoria Climbié inquiry: Report of an inquiry by Lord Laming.* Department of Health.

Part II

Child Development

Therapeutic Play and Maintaining Hope in the Infant Child

Dolores Dooley

Chapter Objectives

At the end of this chapter, you will be able to:

- Describe key developmental tasks and transitions in infancy.
- Explain attachment in relation to the infant–parent relationship.
- Identify key aspects of care which will support optimal development and successful transitions in infancy.
- Consider therapeutic play approaches to enhance infant–parent relationships.

Introduction

Hope is both the earliest and the most indispensable virtue inherent in the state of being alive. .....if life is to be sustained hope must remain, even where confidence is wounded, trust impaired [1, p. 115].

Infancy refers to the period of development from birth through the first year of life, a significant period in the life cycle which is characterised by key developments in physical, social, emotional, and cognitive capabilities. Understanding developmental norms relative to the infant child is important for the provision of optimal care. This chapter focuses on key domains of development of the infant child between the ages of 0–18 months including physical, neurological, attachment and infant play. Incorporating Erikson's psychosocial development stage of trust versus mistrust and Bowlby's secure-base representations, it also includes considerations for nursing and allied health care and the integration of therapeutic play approaches to support infants and their parents as partners.

D. Dooley (✉)
School of Nursing and Midwifery, Deakin University, Geelong, VIC, Australia
e-mail: d.dooley@deakin.edu.au

© The Author(s), under exclusive license to Springer Nature
Switzerland AG 2022
J. A. Parson et al. (eds.), *Integrating Therapeutic Play Into Nursing and Allied Health Practice*, https://doi.org/10.1007/978-3-031-16938-0_6

Child Development and Assessment

Physical Development

Understanding normative measures including expectations for infant growth and development is an important element of health care. Physical growth in infancy is readily visible and measurable and reflects the overall health and wellbeing of the infant child, changes in growth patterns can be a sign of underlying health or development issues. In 2007, the World health Organization (WHO) published international growth standards portraying healthy growth in early childhood [2]. The infants' weight, height, and head circumference are measured according to percentiles which compare each individual infant's measurements with an appropriate age-sex specific growth chart. The standards assess the growth and development of the infant child and are recognised as key indicators of health and wellbeing. Poor weight gain, for example, can be predictive of an underlying medical condition that may require attention.

In Australia, a healthy newborn's birthweight range is between 2500 and 4499 grams [3]. On average, the infant will double their weight by 4 months of age and at 1 year will have tripled their birth weight, their length will increase by about 50% in the first year of life. From 12 months of age, the rate of growth slows and is followed by a steady increase in weight and height until adolescence. Head circumference also increases rapidly during infancy and reflects brain growth, by 12 months the brain is already two-thirds of its adult size [4].

The physiological development that occurs during infancy indicates the significant changes taking place in the brain. At birth the newborn displays a range of reflexes which are essential for adaptation to the extrauterine environment, most of these reflexes disappear over the first year of life as the cerebral cortex develops resulting in an increase in voluntary control of movements [5]. The infant's motor development correlates with increasing development of the nervous system and follows a cephalo-caudal (head to toe) and proximodistal (from midline to outer) sequence [6]. While motor skill milestones progress in an orderly sequence, the age at which each skill is achieved is variable. Exactly when the infant sits, crawls or walks is dependent on several factors including maturation of the neural and muscular system as well as the opportunity to practise motor skills [7]. Parents can be encouraged to notice key stages in motor developmental for example, their infant turning over, sitting, crawling, and standing and can be reassured that their child is progressing as expected for their age or identify when a child requires early intervention.

Psychosocial Development

Erik Erikson (1902–1994), one of the leading figures in the field of psychoanalysis and human development describes fundamental psychosocial stages or crises that the individual must face and resolve to attain healthy development across the lifespan. Regarding infancy, the first crisis of life is basic trust or mistrust. If the infant feels that their caregiver recognises and responds to their essential needs with "*consistency, continuity and sameness of experience"* [1, p. 247], then this develops a sense of trust. Hope is the virtue associated with trust, the infant (and later the child & adult) who can trust that their needs will be met by their caregiver, will develop hope (confidence) in their own ability and learn to trust the self [1]. Conversely, if the infant's physical and/or psychological needs are not met, then the infant will lean towards a mistrust of their world and the self. The capacity to form healthy attachment relationships is closely linked to the experience of trust and hope instilled during infancy.

In essence, infant attachment is the organisation and patterning of behaviours resulting in feelings of trust and closeness to the parent. Attachment theory asserts that biologically based behaviours (crying, smiling, clinging, gazing) support the infant's survival, promote proximity seeking and security, thereby influencing emotional regulation [8]. Ainsworth et al. [9] described attachment styles as secure or insecure. Secure attachment is associated with responsive and consistent caregiving during infancy and contributes to the development of the infant child's self-organising system including their ability to trust. Conversely, insecure attachment is associated with inappropriate or inconsistent care and/or responses from the primary caregiver. The infant does not see the caregiver as a secure base and this may elicit behaviours of anxiety and uncertainty. The secure base concept, central to attachment theory, allows the infant to explore and play knowing the caregiver will be "…. *available, ready to respond when called upon to encourage and perhaps assist, but to intervene actively only when clearly necessary"* [8, p. 11]. The Bowlby–Ainsworth concept of secure (vs. insecure) attachment embraces much of what Erikson meant by trust (vs. mistrust) [10].

A central characteristic of the infant–parent relationships is the development of reciprocal attachment bonds. Brazelton et al. [11] described this reciprocity as the achievement of synchrony. The infant sends cues (cry, smile, gazing, movement) about their readiness to interact, the parent adapts their own behaviour responding to the infant's signals (soothing, cuddling, smiling, feeding). Infant behaviours reinforce the behaviours of the parent, sensitive adjustments made by the mother support the infant to maintain homeostasis and to develop an expanding attention cycle [11]. This reciprocal back and forth between the infant and parent nurtures the development of attachment and emotional growth in the infant child [12]. Creating secure attachment experiences and relationships is important not only for fostering healthy coping skills in the infant but to support brain development. As Siegel [13] states *"… these salient emotional relationships have a direct effect on the development of the domains of mental functioning that serve as our conceptual anchor points: memory, narrative, emotion, representations, and states of mind".*

Neurological Development

Where attention goes, neural firing flows, and neural connection grows [13, p. 41].

Human brain development is a complex and lengthy process beginning shortly after conception and continuing into early adulthood, brain maturation during this period correlates with cognitive, emotional, and social development. The brain develops hierarchically and in a predictable sequence from the most primitive to the most complex parts of the brain, with the lower regions of the brain responsible for physiological homeostasis; the central areas or limbic region responsible for a wide range of mental processes such as emotional activation, motivation, memory, and attachment; and the upper brain structures mediating more complex processes such as language, thought, and reasoning [13]. Brain growth is highly organised, neurons which are specialised nerve cells communicate with each other via synaptic connections and change in response to signals from other parts of the brain, the body or from experiences [14]. Neurons use neurotransmitters (brain chemicals) to communicate across synapses. As the newborn's brain possesses more neurons and connections than is required by an individual, gradual synaptic pruning occurs in infancy and early childhood to remove connections that are not needed, reaching a stable adult level [15]. Experiences to a large degree will determine which synaptic connections will endure and strengthen, and which are selectively eliminated because of inactivity [16].

Greenough et al. [17] distinguish between *experience-expectant* and *experience-dependent* processes guiding brain development. *Experience-expectant* refers to synaptic development that take place when the brain is primed and anticipates the sensory experiences necessary for specific neuronal circuitry organisation. The developing brain "expects" to receive common environmental experiences such as exposure to light to activate the visual cortex or sounds to stimulate the auditory centres in the brain. If these circuits have been deprived of sensory experiences, cell death may occur resulting in lost or reduced functional capacity [13]. *Experience-dependent* refers to new synaptic development triggered entirely by experiences unique to the individual. The experience-dependent nature of brain development highlights the critical importance of relational and social interactions for the infant. Conversely, if the infant is exposed to inappropriate or stressful experiences, the developing brain may not develop as expected. How the brain adapts or changes in response to experiences is called neuroplasticity and the developing brain, particularly during infancy, is remarkably plastic [16]. Indeed, this "large window of plasticity" presents an opportunity for early caregiving relationships to significantly influence the infant's developing brain and support development in key domains [18, p. 328].

Jean Piaget (1896–1980) was a developmental psychologist and the first person to identify stages of cognitive development in children. Piaget proposed four stages of cognitive development, the first stage encompassing birth to 18–24 months is defined as the sensorimotor period during which the infant experiences the world through their senses and motor actions [19]. Piaget believed that cognitive development proceeds through a series of six connected stages within the sensorimotor period where the infant progresses from reflexive behaviours in early infancy to intentional action [20]. In sum, physical, psychosocial (including emotional), neurological, and cognitive development are dynamically linked and work together to foster self-regulation in infancy and beyond [21]. Play is also regarded as essential to development across key domains in infancy. Indeed, Piaget showed that the child acquires knowledge about objects through their action with them, which has been interpreted as learning through play [22].

Play Development

Play is an active and emergent process of engagement with the world, which encompasses exploratory processes. It is repetitive, but not stereotyped, and is spontaneous in nature [23, p. 17].

Infants are social beings. From the moment of birth, the newborn demonstrates that they are indeed active partners in the mother–infant relationship and are already shaping their own environment. Almost immediately, the newborn will selectively attend to the mother's voice and focus on the face, their gaze behaviour signalling a readiness to communicate and to engage in play [12]. From birth, the mother uses baby talk or "motherese", facial expressions and movements, to attract the infant's attention and sustain their interest [24]. These behaviours generate and sustain communicative sequences and help to regulate the infant physiologically and emotionally through sensitive nurturing care. Over the first months, the infant's autonomic nervous system becomes more integrated and stable and from about 4 months, the infant seeks exploratory play [25]. This often takes the form of sensory play (e.g. touch, songs, 'peek-a-boo', or 'this little piggy') which activates a state of co-regulation between the mother-infant as well as triggering the release of oxytocin further enhancing the attachment bond and feelings of trust [24]. Further, neurosensory play interactions, especially touch via gentle massage and stroking, also release neurochemicals (oxytocin, serotonin, and dopamine) in the infant's brain which soothe and calm the infant's nervous system [26]. Exploratory play heightens as the infant begins to crawl about and the desire to explore the world around them increases [20]. The infant who can engage their parent in play and manipulate objects acquires a fundamental belief in their ability to affect their world [27]. Importantly, infants with secure attachments will feel confident in exploring their environment knowing they have a secure base in which to return [28]. The interactions that occur through play reinforce feelings of trust for the infant, as Brown and Vaughan [29] put it, "Play sets the stage for cooperative socialization. It nourishes the roots of trust, empathy, caring and sharing".

Considerations for Nursing and Allied Health Care

…early emotional experiences can have life-long consequences… even though there may be little to be observed in obvious short-term external behaviours ([30], p. 135).

All social emotions affect the brain particularly sadness and fear, the infant sadness implies withdrawal and is associated with physiological stress [20]. When social distress is extreme due to abuse, neglect, or trauma, brain development is disrupted resulting in social, emotional, and cognitive impairment [31]. As Panksepp [30] puts it "*…the larger the sphere of influence of the positive emotions, the more likely is the child to become a productive and happy member of society. The more he or she is influenced by negative emotions, the more the paths toward unhappiness are paved*".

Common Fears and Anxieties

Infants experiencing abnormal social interaction become sad, hesitant, withdrawn, anxious, and vigilant [32]. Berger [20] highlights two kinds of social fear responses typically seen in infancy, stranger wariness, and separation anxiety. Stranger wariness is commonly seen between 7 and 12 months, the infant shows an expression of fear (wrinkled brow, grimace) as a stranger appears. To diminish the impact of stranger fear, gradual introduction to the 'stranger' in the presence of the parent is recommended. Separation fear refers to the infant's anxiety when they are separated from or when the parent leaves the room. The infant will cry "protest" and try and cling to the parent. Separation fear is part of normative development and usually appears between 9 and 14 months then gradually declines. However, when sudden or prolonged separation (such as abandonment) occurs, this may result in life-long susceptibility for sadness, despair, or resentment [30].

Grief and Loss/Death and Dying

The infant child is capable of grief in response to loss, early rejection, or trauma [13, 27]. Bowlby's theory of attachment helps in understanding how the infant construes loss or death of an attachment figure. Secure attachment, that unique relationship between the infant and their parent is protective against social-emotional maladjustment [33]. It is when the parent is perceived as unreachable that "grief" occurs [9, p. 21]. Bowlby observed that infants experienced many of the same reactions as grieving adults when separated from their mothers. The infant losing hope, displays indifference and sadness. A predictable pattern emerges, the infant first engaging in vigorous protest followed sometime later by despair with depression-like symptoms [34, p. 698]. The infant can recover from the loss of an attachment figure if they can rely on an existing caregiver or can attach themselves to another fig [34].

Pain Management

In the 1980s and early 1990s it was common practice for neonates to undergo surgery without anaesthesia or analgesia [35]. It was the voice of a mother who brought neonatal pain to the world's attention. Jill Lawson's baby Jeffrey was born at 26 weeks' gestation in 1986 and underwent surgery for ligation of a patent ductus without any analgesia [36]. Infant pain is a complex phenomenon, being preverbal, assessment of pain is dependent exclusively upon behavioural and physiological responses. Evidence-based behavioural variables are facial expression and diffuse body movement, physiological variables with strong evidence are variability in heart rate and oxygen saturation [37]. Although the ethical imperative to treat infant's pain is beyond question, Harrison [38] argues that there still exists myths, misconceptions, barriers, and knowledge gaps when it comes to using the three key evidenced-based strategies of "breastfeeding, skin-to-skin care (SSC) and sucrose" for infant pain management. Further, she contends that the evidence regarding pain management needs to be put into consistent practice. Although pain assessment is the "fifth" vital sign, Gardner et al. [39] recommend that neonatal pain be viewed as an adverse and traumatic event.

Pain will activate the child's attachment behaviour [40, p. 4] so it is important that the parent is present and supported to help the infant manage their pain and regulate their emotional state. Alongside the three evidenced-based strategies for infant pain management mentioned above, other non-pharmacological interventions that have demonstrated efficacy include: maternal presence; non-nutritive sucking; containment holds; swaddling and developmentally supportive positioning for the smaller infant [41]. In sum, infants do feel pain, it is now known that traumatic experiences in infancy are part of implicit memory, memories that are stored in the body and brain but not recalled through language.

Therapeutic Play Approaches for Clinical Practice

While play occupies a great part of an infant's day, play therapy approaches to support this unique population is a more recent concept. Baldwin et al. [42] defines infant play therapies as "…*informed by the fields of neuroscience and infant mental health, are culturally sensitive, and utilize the therapeutic powers of play to effect positive change for the infant and parental relational system and social environment*".

Several play intervention programmes have stemmed from attachment theory. Benoit [33] asserts that the question we should consider is, *"what is the quality of attachment between this parent and child?"*. The circle of security (COS) is one intervention developed to assist caregivers provide a secure base and enhance infant–parent attachment relationships [43]. The COS graphic [44, p. 110] provides a visual "path to secure attachment" for the parent to help develop their sensitivity and responsiveness to their infant's signal related to the infant moving away from their secure base to explore, and moving back towards their parent's outstretched hands for comfort and soothing. The COS also supports the caregiver's capacity to reflect on their own and the infants' behaviours and interactions as well as how their own developmental history may impact current caregiving behaviours [45]. Several other approaches are available wherein trained play therapists utilise the therapeutic powers of play to optimise outcomes for the infant–parent relationship. For example, FirstPlay ® therapy founded by Dr. Janet Courtney fosters healthy infant–parent relationships by supporting the parent to provide sensitive nurturing care, build trust and increase secure attachment [42]. FirstPlay ® focuses on pre-symbolic play and is underpinned by attachment theory, developmental play therapy, filial therapy, family systems theory, Ericksonian-based storytelling as well as mindfulness and touch therapy [42, p. 84]. Other therapy models to support infant–parent relationships include Theraplay [25] and the embodiment-projection-role model developed by Sue Jennings [46]. The clinician can use therapeutic play approaches within the health care setting to support the infant and their family, for example, through music or singing (e.g. lullabies); touch (massage); playing games (e.g. peek-a-boo); creating a visual environment with mirrors and coloured mobiles or cot toys; using toys to encourage movement (rolling, crawling, kicking). Incorporating therapeutic play can be used to not only assess, support, and maintain the infant's developmental milestones but can be used to empower the parent(s) to be the secure base for their infant. Importantly, the overarching goal of the therapies is to demonstrate empathy, remain hopeful for the infant, and strengthen the parent–infant dyadic relationship.

Parents as Partners

According to Nugent et al. [12], infancy, particularly the early month of life can be "... *the teachable moment par excellence across the lifespan*". The provision of support and positive nurturing experiences during critical periods of brain refinement can have long-lasting implications on the parent–infant relationship and on infant developmental outcomes. Supportive care interventions can be implemented by the clinician and may include modelling social and emotional skills and perspectives; providing practical help and guidance; being attentive towards the infant and modelling this to the parents; complementing parents on their parenting skills; using a nurturing voice and demeanour; encouraging additional attachment figures for the infant; acting as an advocate where necessary; and supporting parents' decision making without enforcing own values or beliefs. The potential cascade of adverse transgenerational transmission of risk can be halted through "...*consistent attitudes of warmth, nurturance, vigorous playfulness, along with a better recognition of how rhythmic-melodic interactions and growth challenges may allow brain systems to flourish*" [30, p. 135].

Considerations for Referral

The infants' early relationship experiences influence the developing brain, thus, the need for early identification and interventions to support emotional engagement and attachment. Screening should commence antenatally and appropriate referrals made (e.g. for anxiety/depression; drugs/alcohol). Similarly, in the postnatal period, it is essential to screen for mood disorders or any infant–parent relationship or interactional difficulties and refer accordingly.

Chapter Summary

Infancy is a fascinating period of human development, the changes that occur across the developmental domains during this period are significant and have implications across the life span. Positive nurturing experiences are critical for optimal organisation and development of the brain particularly during infancy. Early caregiving matters, a secure attachment fosters trust and facilitates self-regulation in the infant.

Conversely, mistrust or an insecure base brings about feelings of despair and hopelessness. The infant brain displays great plasticity—this is where the *hope* lies. Supporting positive infant–parent relational experiences and incorporating therapeutic play can enhance brain development and set the stage for healthy future development. In sum, it is essential that clinicians are aware of potential risks that may impact the infant especially in relation to infant–parent attachment. Then prioritising the creation of safe, nurturing, and playful environments and including parents as partners thereby promoting and maintaining hope in the infant child.

Reflective Questions and Activities

1. Observe infants in public places, for example, the supermarket, playground, on public transport. From your observations, consider body size, gross and fine motor skills, play development and interactions—are they 'typical'?
2. Discuss the parallels between Erikson's trust verse mistrust and Bowlby's secure-base model of attachment.
3. Review one or more of the therapeutic play approaches mentioned above and consider how you could incorporate aspects of these therapies into your clinical practice.

Additional Resources

https://www.zerotothree.org/resources/156-brain-wonders-nurturing-healthy-brain-development-from-birth
https://www.startingblocks.gov.au/other-resources/factsheets/brain-development-in-children/
https://www.aaimh.org.au/

References

1. Erikson, E. H. (1964). *Insight and responsibility : lectures on the ethical implications of psychoanalytic insight* ([First edition] ed.) [Bibliographies]. W.W. Norton. Retrieved from https://search.ebscohost.com/login.aspx?direct=true&db=cat00097a&AN=deakin.b1042934&authtype=sso&custid=deakin&site=eds-live&scope=site
2. WHO. (2007). *Child growth standards*. Retrieved from https://www.who.int/tools/child-growth-standards/standards
3. Health, A. I. o., & Welfare. (2021). *Australia's mothers and babies*. Retrieved from https://www.aihw.gov.au/reports/mothers-babies/australias-mothers-babies
4. Pillitteri, A., & Haley, C. (2016). Pillitteri's child and family health nursing in Australia and New Zealand (2nd ed.) [Bibliographies]. Lippincott Williams & Wilkins. Retrieved from https://search.ebscohost.com/login.aspx?direct=true&db=cat00097a&AN=deakin.b4687328&authtype=sso&custid=deakin&site=eds-live&scope=site, http://ezproxy.deakin.edu.au/login?url=https://ovidsp.ovid.com/ovidweb.cgi?T=JS&NEWS=n&CSC=Y&PAGE=booktext&D=books&AN=02118362$&XPATH=/PG(0)&EPUB=Y

5. Brazelton, T. B., & Nugent, J. K. (2011). *Neonatal behavioral assessment scale* (Fourth edition. ed.) [Bibliographies]. Mac Keith Press. Retrieved from https://ezproxy.deakin.edu.au/login?url=https://search.ebscohost.com/login.aspx?direct=true&db=cat00097a&AN=deakin.b2681598&authtype=sso&custid=deakin&site=eds-live&scope=site, http://ezproxy.deakin.edu.au/login?url=http://search.ebscohost.com/login.aspx?direct=true&scope=site&db=e000xww&AN=503755, http://ezproxy.deakin.edu.au/login?url=http://ebookcentral.proquest.com/lib/deakin/detail.action?docID=3329164

6. Adolph, K. E., Vereijken, B., & Denny, M. A. (1998). Learning to crawl. *Child Development, 69*(5), 1299–1312. https://doi.org/10.1111/j.1467-8624.1998.tb06213.x

7. Adolph, K. E., & Franchak, J. M. (2017). The development of motor behavior [article]. *WIREs. Cognitive Science, 8*(1/2) n/a-N.PAG. https://doi.org/10.1002/wcs.1430

8. Bowlby, J. (1988). *A secure base : Parent-child attachment and healthy human development* [bibliographies]. Basic Books. Retrieved from https://search.ebscohost.com/login.aspx?direct=true&db=cat00097a&AN=deakin.b1362081&authtype=sso&custid=deakin&site=eds-live&scope=site.

9. Ainsworth, M. D. S., Blehar, M., Waters, E., & Wall, S. N. (1978). *Patterns of attachment : a psychological study of the strange situation [bibliographies]*. Lawrence Erlbaum Associates. Retrieved from https://search.ebscohost.com/login.aspx?direct=true&db=cat00097a&AN=deakin.b1060314&authtype=sso&custid=deakin&site=eds-live&scope=site

10. Pittman, J. F., Keiley, M. K., Kerpelman, J. L., & Vaughn, B. E. (2011). Attachment, identity, and intimacy: Parallels between Bowlby's and Erikson's paradigms. *Journal of Family Theory & Review, 3*(1), 32–46. Retrieved from https://search.ebscohost.com/login.aspx?direct=true&db=edb&AN=65007932&authtype=sso&custid=deakin&site=eds-live&scope=site

11. Brazelton, T. B., Koslowski, B., & Main, M. (1974). The origins of reciprocity: The early mother-infant interaction. In *The effect of the infant on its caregiver.* (pp. xxiv, 264-xxiv, 264). Wiley-Interscience.

12. Nugent, J. K., Keeker, C. H., Minear, S., Johnson, L. C., & Blanchard, Y. (2007). *Understanding newborn behavior and early relationships : The newborn behavioral observations (NBO) system handbook [bibliographies]*. P.H. Brookes. Retrieved from https://search.ebscohost.com/login.aspx?direct=true&db=cat00097a&AN=deakin.b2281018&authtype=sso&custid=deakin&site=eds-live&scope=site

13. Siegel, D. J. A (2020). *The developing mind : How relationships and the brain interact to shape who we are* (3rd ed) [Bibliographies]. The Guilford Press. Retrieved from https://search.ebscohost.com/login.aspx?direct=true&db=cat00097a&AN=deakin.b4372274&authtype=sso&custid=deakin&site=eds-live&scope=site, http://ezproxy.deakin.edu.au/login?url=https://ebookcentral.proquest.com/lib/deakin/detail.action?docID=6172778

14. Blackburn, S. T. (2013). *Maternal, fetal, & neonatal physiology : a clinical perspective* (4th ed.). Elsevier Saunders. Retrieved from https://search.ebscohost.com/login.aspx?direct=true&db=cat00097a&AN=deakin.b2666330&authtype=sso&custid=deakin&site=eds-live&scope=site

15. Kolb, B., & Whishaw, I. Q. (2009). *Fundamentals of human neuropsychology.* 6th edn. [Bibliographies]. Worth Publisher. Retrieved from https://search.ebscohost.com/login.aspx?direct=true&db=cat00097a&AN=deakin.b2341692&authtype=sso&custid=deakin&site=eds-live&scope=site

16. Kolb, B., & Gibb, R. (2011). Brain plasticity and behaviour in the developing brain. *Journal of the Canadian academy of child and adolescent psychiatry = journal de l'Academie canadienne de psychiatrie de l'enfant et de l'adolescent, 20*(4), 265–276. Retrieved from https://pubmed.ncbi.nlm.nih.gov/22114608, https://www.ncbi.nlm.nih.gov/pmc/articles/PMC3222570/

17. Greenough, W. T., Black, J. E., & Wallace, C. S. (1987). Experience and brain development [Article]. *Child Development, 58*(3), 539. https://doi.org/10.2307/1130197

18. Bernier, A., Carlson, S. M., & Whipple, N. (2010). From external regulation to self-regulation: Early parenting precursors of young children's executive functioning. *Child Development, 81*(1), 326–339. https://doi.org/10.1111/j.1467-8624.2009.01397.x

19. Piaget, J., & Cook, M. (1952). *The origins of intelligence in children* [Electronic]. W.W. Norton. Retrieved from https://search.ebscohost.com/login.aspx?direct=true&db=cat00097a&AN=de

akin.b3347328&authtype=sso&custid=deakin&site=eds-live&scope=site; http://ezproxy.dea-kin.edu.au/login?url=https://search.ebscohost.com/direct.asp?db=pzh&jid=200710742

20. Berger, K. S. A (2019). *The developing person through childhood and adolescence* (Eleventh edition. ed.) [Bibliographies]. Macmillan Learning. Retrieved from https://search.ebscohost.com/login.aspx?direct=true&db=cat00097a&AN=deakin.b4405945&authtype=sso&custid=deakin&site=eds-live&scope=site, http://ezproxy.deakin.edu.au/login?url=https://ebookcen-tral.proquest.com/lib/deakin/detail.action?docID=6234965

21. Rosenblum, K. L., Dayton, C. J., & Muzik, M. (2009). Infant social and emotional devel-opment. In C. H. Zeanah (Ed.), *Handbook of infant mental health* (3rd ed., pp. 80–103). Guilford Press. Retrieved from. Retrieved from https://search.ebscohost.com/login.aspx?dir-ect=true&db=cat00097a&AN=deakin.b3539014&authtype=sso&custid=deakin&site=eds-live&scope=site, http://ezproxy.deakin.edu.au/login?url=http://ebookcentral.proquest.com/lib/deakin/detail.action?docID=454796

22. Belsky, J., & Most, R. K. (1981). From exploration to play: A cross-sectional study of infant free play behavior. *Developmental Psychology, 17*(5), 630–639. https://doi.org/10.1037/0012-1649.17.5.630

23. Hedges, J. H., Adolph, K. E., Amso, D., Bavelier, D., Fiez, J. A., Krubitzer, L., McAuley, J. D., Newcombe, N. S., Fitzpatrick, S. M., & Ghajar, J. (2013). Play, attention, and learning: How do play and timing shape the development of attention and influence classroom learning? *Annals of the New York Academy of Sciences, 1292*, 1–20. https://doi.org/10.1111/nyas.12154

24. Dissanayake, E. (2017). Ethology, interpersonal neurobiology, and play: Insights into the evolutionary origin of the arts [article]. *American Journal of Play, 9*(2), 143–168. Retrieved from https://search.ebscohost.com/login.aspx?direct=true&db=a9h&AN=123136212&site=eds-live&scope=site

25. Booth, P. B., Lender, D., & Lindaman, S. (2018). Playing with someone who loves you: Creating safety and joyful parent-child connection with theraplay. In T. Marks-Tarlow, M. F. Solomon, & D. J. Siegel (Eds.), *Play and creativity in psychotherapy* (1st ed., pp. 217–241). W.W Norton & Company. W.W Norton & Company. Retrieved from https://search.ebscohost.com/login.aspx?direct=true&db=cat00097a&AN=deakin.b3746535&authtype=sso&custid=deakin&site=eds-live&scope=site

26. Schwartzenberger, K. (2020). Neurosensory play in the infant-parent dyad. In J. A. Courtney (Ed.), Infant play therapy : Foundations, models, programs, and practice (pp. 37–49). Routledge. Retrieved from https://search.ebscohost.com/login.aspx?direct=true&db=cat00097a&AN=deakin.b4347152&authtype=sso&custid=deakin&site=eds-live&scope=site, http://ezproxy.deakin.edu.au/login?url=https://ebookcentral.proquest.com/lib/deakin/detail.action?docID=6132272

27. Phillips, D., & Shonkoff, J. P. (2000). *From neurons to neighborhoods : The science of early childhood development [Bibliographies]*. National Academy Press. Retrieved from https://search.ebscohost.com/login.aspx?direct=true&db=cat00097a&AN=deakin.b1945496&authtype=sso&custid=deakin&site=eds-live&scope=site

28. Gillespie, L., & Hunter, A. (2011). Creating healthy attachments to the babies in your care [research-article]. *YC Young Children, 66*(5), 62–63. Retrieved from https://search.ebscohost.com/login.aspx?direct=true&db=edsjsr&AN=edsjsr.42730775&authtype=sso&custid=deakin&site=eds-live&scope=site

29. Brown, S. L., & Vaughan, C. C. (2009). *Play : how it shapes the brain, opens the imagination, and invigorates the soul* [Bibliographies]. Avery. Retrieved from https://search.ebscohost.com/login.aspx?direct=true&db=cat00097a&AN=deakin.b3537979&authtype=sso&custid=deakin&site=eds-live&scope=site. http://ezproxy.deakin.edu.au/login?url=http://ebookcentral.pro-quest.com/lib/deakin/detail.action?docID=618796.

30. Panksepp, J. (2001). The long-term psychobiological consequences of infant emotions: Prescriptions for the twenty-first century [article]. *Infant Mental Health Journal, 22*(1/2), 132–173. https://doi.org/10.1002/1097-0355(200101/04)22:1<132::AID-IMHJ5>3.0.CO;2-9

31. Felitti, V. J., Anda, R. F., Nordenberg, D., Williamson, D. F., Spitz, A. M., Edwards, V., Koss, M. P., & Marks, J. S. (2019). Relationship of childhood abuse and household dysfunction to

many of the leading causes of death in adults: The adverse childhood experiences (ACE) study [article]. *American Journal of Preventive Medicine, 56*(6), 774–786. https://doi.org/10.1016/j.amepre.2019.04.001

32. Tronick, E. (2014). Typical and atypical development: Peek-a-boo and blind selection. In K. Brandt, B. D. Perry, S. Seligman, E. Tronick, & T. B. Brazelton (Eds.), *Infant and early childhood mental health: Core concepts and clinical practice* (1st ed., pp. 55–70). American Psychiatric Association Publishing. Retrieved from https://ezproxy.deakin.edu.au/login?url=https://search.ebscohost.com/login.aspx?direct=true&db=nlebk&AN=1594708&authtype=sso&custid=deakin&site=eds-live&scope=site

33. Benoit, D. (2004). Infant-parent attachment: Definition, types, antecedents, measurement and outcome [review]. *Paediatrics and Child Health, 9*(8), 541–545. https://doi.org/10.1093/pch/9.8.541

34. Sigelman, C. K. A De George-Walker, L., Cunial, K., & Rider, E. A. (2019). *Life span human development* (Third Australian and New Zealand edition. ed.) [Bibliographies]. Cengage Learning Australia. Retrieved from https://search.ebscohost.com/login.aspx?direct=true&db=cat00097a&AN=deakin.b4118727&authtype=sso&custid=deakin&site=eds-live&scope=site, http://ezproxy.deakin.edu.au/login?url=https://ebookcentral.proquest.com/lib/deakin/detail.action?docID=6335527, http://ezproxy.deakin.edu.au/login?url=https://ebookcentral.proquest.com/lib/deakin/detail.action?docID=5723228

35. Anand, K. J. S. M. D., & Hickey, P. M. (1987). Pain and its effects in the human neonate and fetus. *The New England Journal of Medicine, 317*(21), 1321–1329. Retrieved from http://ezproxy.deakin.edu.au/login?url=https://www.proquest.com/scholarly-journals/pain-effects-human-neonate-fetus/docview/1884545878/se-2?accountid=10445. https://library.deakin.edu.au/resserv?genre=article&issn=00284793&title=The+New+England+Journal+of+Medicine&volume=317&issue=21&date=1987-11-19&atitle=Pain+and+Its+Effects+in+the+Human+Neonate+and+Fetus&spage=1321&aulast=Anand&sid=ProQ:ProQ%3Ahealthcompleteshell&isbn=&jtitle=The+New+England+Journal+of+Medicine&btitle=&id=doi:

36. Lawson, J. R. (1986). LETTERS. *Birth, 13*(2), 124–125. https://doi.org/10.1111/j.1523-536X.1986.tb01024.x

37. Hatfield, L. A., & Ely, E. A. (2015). Measurement of acute pain in infants: a review of behavioral and physiological variables. *Biological Research for Nursing, 17*(1), 100–111. https://doi.org/10.1177/1099800414531448

38. Harrison, D. (2021). Pain management for infants – Myths, misconceptions, barriers; knowledge and knowledge gaps [review article]. *Journal of Neonatal Nursing, 27*(5), 313–316. https://doi.org/10.1016/j.jnn.2020.12.004

39. Gardner, S. L., Hines, M. E., & Agarwal, R. (2021). Pain and pain relief. In S. L. Gardner, B. S. Carter, M. E. Hines, & S. Niermeyer (Eds.), *Merenstein & Gardner's handbook of neonatal intensive care* (9th ed., pp. 273–333). Elsevier. Retrieved from https://search.ebscohost.com/login.aspx?direct=true&db=cat00097a&AN=deakin.b4451663&authtype=sso&custid=deakin&site=eds-live&scope=site, http://ezproxy.deakin.edu.au/login?url=https://ebookcentral.proquest.com/lib/deakin/detail.action?docID=6039438

40. Bowlby, J., & Holmes, J. (2005). *A Secure Base*. Taylor & Francis Group. Retrieved from http://ebookcentral.proquest.com/lib/deakin/detail.action?docID=1075270

41. Altimier, L., & Phillips, R. (2016). The neonatal integrative developmental care model: Advanced clinical applications of the seven Core measures for neuroprotective family-centered developmental care. *Newborn and Infant Nursing Reviews, 16*(4), 230–244. https://doi.org/10.1053/j.nainr.2016.09.030

42. Baldwin, K., Velasquez, M., & Courtney, J. A. (2020). FirstPlay ®therapy strengthens the attachment relationship between a mother with perinatal depression and her infant. In J. A. Courtney (Ed.), *Infant play therapy: Foundations, models, programs, and practice* (pp. 83–100). Routledge. Retrieved from https://search.ebscohost.com/login.aspx?direct=true&db=cat00097a&AN=deakin.b4347152&authtype=sso&custid=deakin&site=eds-live&scope=site. http://ezproxy.deakin.edu.au/login?url=https://ebookcentral.proquest.com/lib/deakin/detail.action?docID=6132272

43. Powell, B., Cooper, G., Hoffman, K., & Marvin, R. S. (2009). The circle of security. In C. H. Zeanah (Ed.), *Handbook of infant mental health* (3rd ed., pp. 450–467). Guilford Press. Retrieved from https://search.ebscohost.com/login.aspx?direct=true&db=cat0009 7a&AN=deakin.b3539014&authtype=sso&custid=deakin&site=eds-live&scope=site. http://ezproxy.deakin.edu.au/login?url=http://ebookcentral.proquest.com/lib/deakin/detail. action?docID=454796

44. Marvin, R., Cooper, G., Hoffman, K., & Powell, B. (2002). The circle of security project: Attachment-based intervention with caregiver-pre-school child dyads. *Attachment and Human Development, 4*(1), 107–124. https://doi.org/10.1080/14616730252982491

45. Zeanah, C. H., Berlin, L. J., & Boris, N. W. (2011). Practitioner review: Clinical applications of attachment theory and research for infants and young children [article]. *Journal of Child Psychology & Psychiatry, 52*(8), 819–833. https://doi.org/10.1111/j.1469-7610.2011.02399.x

46. Prendiville, E. (2021). The EPR informed psychotherapist. In E. Prendiville & J. Parson (Eds.), *Clinical applications of the therapeutic powers of play: Case studies in child and adolescent psychotherapy* (1st ed.). Routledge. Retrieved from https://search.ebscohost.com/login.aspx? direct=true&db=cat00097a&AN=deakin.b4446916&authtype=sso&custid=deakin&site=eds-live&scope=site. http://ezproxy.deakin.edu.au/login?url=https://ebookcentral.proquest.com/lib/deakin/detail.action?docID=6465154

Therapeutic Play, Volition, and the Toddler

Rhiannon Breguet

Objectives

At the end of this chapter, you will be able to:

- Describe the key milestones in development for children aged between 18 months and 3 years.
- Describe Erikson's stage of autonomy verses shame and doubt and how this applies to the toddler.
- Consider the use of therapeutic play to engage the toddler in a developmentally sensitive manner and identify play and environmental considerations that may assist in engaging the toddler in the health care setting.
- Consider the role of attachment and engaging parents as partners when working with toddlers.

Introduction

The more slowly trees grow at first, the sounder they are at the core, and I think the same is true for human beings—Henry David Thoreau

Nursing and allied health care professionals are in a unique position to support toddlers through challenging health care experiences. This chapter considers caring for children, aged between 18 months and 3 years as they navigate Erikson's psychosocial developmental stage of autonomy versus shame and doubt. Child development refers to the sequence of development that occurs from birth to the

R. Breguet (✉)
Geelong Play Therapy, Casual Academic, Deakin University, Burwood, VIC, Australia
e-mail: rhiannon.breguet@deakin.edu.au

© The Author(s), under exclusive license to Springer Nature
Switzerland AG 2022
J. A. Parson et al. (eds.), *Integrating Therapeutic Play Into Nursing and Allied Health Practice*, https://doi.org/10.1007/978-3-031-16938-0_7

beginning of adulthood. While each child is unique, children typically move through comparable paths of development. It is strongly influenced by a range of factors including genetic factors, prenatal experiences, the environment, and the child–caregiver attachment relationship. Child development is dramatic, rapid, and incredibly complex within the first 2 years of life. During this developmental stage toddlers are energetic, curious, enjoy exploration via their senses, and exploring their physical skills [1]. Child development can be positively influenced by physical and emotional safety and can be slowed by various negative experiences such as trauma, abuse, or neglect [2]. An understanding of child development provides the health care professional with knowledge that can be used to engage the child and tailor interventions to a child's chronological age and developmental stage.

Child Development and Assessment

Physical Development

Physical development encompasses changes in physical growth. Over the course of the first few years of life children grow in spurts, where they experience periods of rapid growth followed by periods of stability. Children typically by the age of three, experience an increase in both gross and fine motor skills [3]. Gross motor skills involve large body movements that enable toddlers to explore their environment independently. Toddlers typically commence walking by the age of 2 years and may have commenced running and climbing, reaching almost full mobility, but lacking preciseness in coordination. By this time a toddler's mobility sharply increases and follows a predicative trajectory. From an infant first learning to move their head and hold it steady, to rolling over, sitting up, standing with support, and then independently walking, leaping, and kicking with somewhat accuracy [3]. While growth occurs in spurts, it is slower in the toddler in comparison to the first 2 years of life. In this stage the toddlers' body portions continue to transform through the development of their torso and legs [2].

Fine motor skills allow children to manipulate small objects and control their hands and arms. Throughout the first year of growth infants increase their finger and hand coordination and by 2 years of age they are more proficient with a pincer grip, and self-care skills such as eating with their hands or with utensils. They are learning to turn pages of books and manipulate small toys. This increase in dexterity permits selective engagement with their environment due to movements becoming more controlled and deliberate [3]. Toddlers have an unflappable desire to explore and exert control over their bodies and the world around them. They begin to show interest in toilet training and display an increased curiosity in their bodies. During this time, they possess few inhibitions around nudity, and show an increased interest in their genitals leading to self-exploration and differentiating between genders [2].

Neurological Development

Neurological development is how the brain grows and integrates cognitive and emotional capabilities. By the age of three, children have experienced tremendous neurological development, accompanied by a decline in physical growth and an increase in cognitive capabilities. Research has found that a child's environment, attachment relationships, and experiences within childhood impact the formation of the brain [1, 2]. Brain development occurs sequentially in a 'bottom up' fashion from those parts of the brain responsible for primitive, survival functions, such as breathing, to the 'top' parts of the brain responsible for more complex functions such as judgement and decision making [4]. Siegal and Payne Bryson [5] developed a simplified model of the brain—the upstairs downstairs brain—based on the analogy of a two-story house. The downstairs house is the engine of the body, responsible for bodily functions such as regulating arousal, body temperature, heart rate, beathing, reflexes, and the flight, fight or freeze response. Like the downstairs of a house, where the kitchen, living room and bathroom are located to service basic needs, this part of the brain accommodates the most primitive section of the brain, the brainstem, which is the most developed part of the brain at birth [5].

The upstairs part of the brain is the most complex part of the brain and houses the cortex. This is where thinking, creativity, planning, decision making, empathy, problem solving, and a sense of self reside. This part of the brain makes us human, is the most evolved part of the brain, and the very last to mature developing into adulthood [2, 6]. For toddlers, while the lower parts of the brain are consolidating, their upstairs brain remains largely under construction, which can explain why toddlers find it difficult to control their impulses. Toddlers need the assistance of others to help them become aware of and regulate their emotions and impulses [2]. The upstairs and downstairs need to work in unison, and adults can assist children to integrate these parts of the brain. Both parents and health care professionals can support the integration of the toddler's brain by having age and developmentally informed expectations around the toddler's behaviour. Toddlers cannot be expected to always make good decisions and regulate their big emotions as their brains are still under construction and these skills are still in development. Toddlers need the help of an adult brain to help them regulate through connection and co-regulation and the provision of regulatory activities such as sensory motor activities that involve moving their body or engaging in sensory play [5].

Psychosocial Development

Children require an array of social skills and social intelligence to be able to create, nurture, and develop loving intimate relationships into adulthood. Eric Erikson believed that humans develop identity through their environment and social interactions and identified eight stages of psychosocial development. Children need to develop through each stage, solving challenges to progress to the next stage. Without this, children may not have all the tools to navigate challenging life events.

If a stage is missed or underdeveloped, children may require support to revisit and resolve each stage. In the first stage of development, trust versus mistrust, the infant child is dependent on their caregivers for comfort and protection. In toddlerhood, children move into the second stage of psychosocial development which occurs from 10 months to 2 or 3 years of age. This stage of development is titled autonomy verses shame and doubt and is characterised by exploration, where the toddler wishes to discover their world, seek self-expression and increase their autonomy [7]. Toddlers who successfully traverse this stage of development achieve greater self-control and an ability to separate from their caregivers, which in turn results in the psychological strength or virtue called will. Toddlers who struggle within this stage may devlop feeling of shame, insecurity, lack boundaries, become risk adverse, or rigid in behaviour. If a toddler masters this stage, they develop confidence in their abilities and achievements and develop a sense of self-worth which leads to the capacity to develop positive relationships, mutual respect, and free expression [2, 7].

While toddlers are developing a greater sense of self-control and seeking autonomy from their caregivers, the attachment relationship is still vital at this stage of development. A positive attachment relationship is helpful in the activation of a child's emotional and social intelligence allowing them to learn, be attentive, reflect, plan, regulate their emotions, be empathic and problem solve. The Circle of Security (COS) provides a model for attachment that explores the role of the caregiver as safe haven and secure base. This model acknowledges the core need of a child for exploration as part of the attachment relationship which fits with Erickson's second stage of psychosocial development, characterised by exploration and volition. Toddlers who are provided with secure attachment have greater capacity to explore their environment, leading to greater exploration of their world, themselves, and increased autonomy [8].

Play Development

Play is fundamental for children, it influences their physical, social, cognitive, and emotional well-being. Play is also important to a child's brain development. It is through play that children from an early age learn and engage with the world around them. For parents, play also provides an opportunity to engage with their children in a meaningful way and provides insight into a child's inner world. For the health care professional, play can be used to engage children at an age-appropriate development level [9].

Play is a sequentially developing ability and can be aligned with a toddler's age and stage. During this stage two-year-olds show enjoyment in their body's movements. They display an increased ability to show sequences within their play, enjoy interactive signing games, mirroring sounds and gestures, and begin to try out role play related to activities such as feeding a baby doll. They partake in mainly solitary play whereby they prefer to play on their own and spectator play, whereby they watch others play but do not interact. Solitary play facilities a toddler's development in imagination and creativity. It also builds self-esteem, attention, increases curiosity, social skills, and language [10]. Play materials at this stage may include toys that move, dolls and teddies, blocks, large crayons, water and sand play. By the age of three the toddler includes more symbolic and interactive aspects to their play. They may begin to discover imaginary creatures, increase the depth of their role play and project their desires onto another play companion. Most toddlers' play is characterised by their real-life experiences and dramatic role play continues to increase in the context of one-on-one relationships. They also have commenced parallel play whereby the toddler will play next to or near another child. Play materials enjoyed by a three-year-old may include doll accessories, stuffed animals, messy play, drawing, and materials that they can sort [10].

Play materials are important as they aid in the expression of a child's inner self, and assist the toddler in conveying abstract concepts, such as emotion [2]. However, a toddler's play is not activated by play materials alone and can be enhanced by an engaged adult in relational experiences and physical play interactions. These play experiences lay the foundation for self-regulation, resiliency, and the ability to manage stress. Physical social play or rough and tumble play also has an important place in toddlerhood due to its positive effect on brain development and self-regulation. Other benefits include learning social rules, the stimulation of anti-stress chemicals, decreased impulsivity, and increased self-esteem. Not to mention it is fun [1].

Considerations for Nursing and Allied Health Care

Children love and want to be loved and they very much prefer the joy of accomplishment to the triumph of hateful failure. Do not mistake a child for his symptom.—Erik Erickson

Working with children in early childhood involves understanding the importance of the physical and psychosocial tasks children engage in, including the development of social skills, language, and autonomy [9]. Children within this developmental stage often display tantrums, non-cooperation, and irritability. It is important that expectations around typical development are conveyed to families [2]. Medical information can be tailored to a child's developmental stage to help children prepare for procedures, recover from medical interventions, and/or make sense of their diagnosis. For example, by creating a social story or a picture book that provides a narrative of a child's medical intervention. A transitional object, for example a favourite toy or blanket, may also support a child's feeling of safety and reduce stress.

Common Fears and Anxieties

A common fear at this age is separation anxiety. This is a fear of being separated from parents or caregivers. Toddlers may display their distress by crying and clinging to their parent. Separation anxiety is a common aspect of child development that commences in infancy and typically dissipates throughout early childhood. Fear of strangers may also occur within this developmental stage and typically diminishers around 2 years of age, however, can continue depending on a toddler's temperament [11]. When bonding chemicals in the brain are activated, this leads to reduced anxiety, fear, and stress. Therefore, it is optimal to ensure that a toddler has access to a parent or caregiver who can provide comfort during times of stress, such as medical procedures.

Pain Management

A child's developmental capacities are a major mediating factor in how a child interprets a painful medical event. The younger the child, the less likely it is that they will be able to make a conscious connection between a previously frightening or painful medical experience and states of hyperarousal, dysregulated behaviours and moods [12]. Health care professionals can assist toddlers by providing activities that can increase brain well-being chemicals and reduce stress hormones. This may include activities such as massage, water play, sensory play, touch objects, warmth, movement, and rocking. These activities can assist in releasing chemicals in the brain that help the child to regulate [1].

Therapeutic Play Approaches for Clinical Practice

> *The playing adult steps sideward into another reality; the playing child advances forward to a new stage of mastery—Eric Erickson*

Toddlers receiving health care require age-appropriate communication to ensure a positive health care experience. Quite often, toddlers may be afraid or anxious about visiting health care settings and this can be eased by considering the environment and how toddlers and parents are engaged in the health care setting.

Environmental Considerations

First impressions matter. It is essential toddlers experience an environment that feels safe and comfortable. In a clinical setting consider creating a 'holding' space in the waiting area to support a smooth transition into the treating room. Consider the noise level, smells, and lighting, ensure that these are of a soothing nature and not overstimulating. Decorate the room with fun playful items and consider providing activities for toddlers that include sensory objects, books and pretend play objects. If possible, make sure they can be easily sanitised. In the treatment room—to assist in engagement and cooperation, again consider the space, ensure safety, and a comfortable quiet environment. Age-appropriate playful objects that toddlers can hold may also assist the child to feel more comfortable and serve as a distraction during assessment or medical procedures. An environment that provides engagement through, cognitive (thinking), physical (movement), social (relational), and sensory (stimulating), has been found to reduce stress chemicals in the brain, reduce anxiety, develop positive attachment, aid memory, increase social skills, and enhance self-regulation [1].

Engaging the Child

Ensure that you allow the toddler time to 'warm up'. Try not to rush them and provide time and space to allow them to warm to you as a health care professional and to the environment. Toddlers attempt to read facial and body expressions, therefore make eye contact and get physically at their level to ensure that you do not tower above them. This can convey a deep respect to the toddler. Quietly introduce yourself, convey warmth and friendliness, humour can be advantageous where appropriate. Children at this stage find humour related to poo and fluctuance incredibly hilarious. So, use your creative flow and unleash your crazy funny [1]. Engage in conversation, be well versed in toddler interests. This can facilitate a relationship of trust, reduce anxiety, and increase rapport. Be curious and consider how you use your facial expressions and tone of voice to communicate care to the child. Tracking can also assist in engaging a toddler. You may track or verbalise what you observe the child doing or looking at, such as 'You're looking around the room to see what is in here'.

Toddlers can be unsure about what to anticipate during a medical consultation and may tend to make their own assumptions on what is going to happen. Proving a toddler with a narrative may help dispel any illogical or scary scenarios they may have created in their mind. Toddlers are still developing their language, so this should be simplified. For example, 'today I am going check your tummy, listen to your heart and see how tall you are. At the end I will talk with your mum and then it will be time to go home'. This provides the toddler with a clear structure, helping them to prepare for what is going to happen next and reduce the fear of the unknown. You may also demonstrate procedures with the help of a doll or toy. You may invite the toddler to be an 'assistant' as toddlers enjoy a 'job', it makes them feel special and in control. They could also have access to a special doctor's coat, hat, or a sticker badge to make this more playful.

It is also important to convey empathy and unconditional positive regard (UPR). As mentioned, a toddler does not yet have a fully wired brain and is still learning to control their emotional and physical impulses. A toddler cannot speak or listen carefully when they are distressed and require the help of an adult to navigate stressful experiences. Providing empathy and UPR can assist a toddler to make sense of uncertain experiences and develop new neural networks, where the brain practises reflecting instead of reacting [1].

Parents as Partners

Effective communication with parents is essential for creating a positive experience for the toddler. It is fundamental that early childhood interventions are rooted in the child–parent/caregiver relationship. Not only to do toddlers need to be provided with empathy, patience, and UPR, so do parents and caregivers. Parents and caregivers want to protect and avoid distress to their toddler. Sometimes parents can be as anxious as their child. Toddlers can also pick up on parental distress and emotional atmospheres [1]. If a parent seems overwhelmed themselves, consider speaking with the parent separately from the child to avoid the children being present during stressful or difficult conversations.

Considerations for Referral

Within the health care setting children may need to be referred for specialists therapeutic intervention if there are concerns for the parent–toddler relationship, when there are concerns for a child's development, or where children may have experienced medical trauma or demonstrate indicators of psychological distress.

Chapter Summary

We don't stop playing because we grow old: We grow old because we stop playing—George Bernard Shaw

To best support toddlers and their families, professionals require an understanding of child development. Working with toddlers within this stage of development can be challenging and rewarding, they can experience big emotions, and need carefully considered regulatory and relational experiences. Health care professionals who utilise playful approaches can engage toddlers in a developmentally sensitive manner. An awareness of the importance of promoting play with families and service providers is vital in the delivery of therapeutically sensitive health care. When health care professionals achieve the cooperation and attention of a toddler, the anxiety levels for both the toddler and the caregiver are decreased, which may in turn lead to improved patient outcomes.

Reflective Questions and Activities

- How might an understanding of the upstairs and downstairs brain help you to better understand the toddler?
- Examine the physical space within a medical setting (e.g. the waiting room or treatment room). Attempt to see the space through the eyes of a toddler. Are there

changes that could be made to assist a toddler to feel comfortable and relaxed? What toys might be appropriate to include for a toddler within this space?
- What as some ideas for developmentally sensitive toys or play activities you could use with a toddler during a medical assessment?

Additional Resources

- **Website**—The Raising Kids website has fantastic information on child development as well as resources for parents. https://raisingchildren.net.au/preschoolers/play-learning/active-play/rough-play-guide

References

1. Sunderland, M. (2006). *What every parent needs to know* (2nd ed.). London.
2. Ray, D. C. (2015). *A therapist's guide to child development: The extraordinarily normal years.* Routledge.
3. Berger, K. S. (2011). *The developing person through childhood and adolescence* (8th ed.). Worth.
4. Perry, B. (2009). Examining child maltreatment through a neurodevelopmental lens: Clinical applications of the neurosequential model of therapeutics. *Journal of Loss & Trauma, 14*(4), 240–255. https://doi.org/10.1080/15325020903004350
5. Siegel, D. J., & Payne Bryson, T. (2011). *The whole-brain child: 12 revolutionary strategies to nurture your child's developing mind.* Bantam Books.
6. Music, G. (2016). *Nurturing natures: Attachment and Children's emotional, sociocultural and brain development* (2nd ed.). Routledge, Taylor & Francis Group.
7. Erickson, E. (1963). *Childhood and society.* Norton.
8. Hoffman, K. T., Marvin, R. S., Cooper, G., & Powell, B. (2006). Changing toddlers' and preschoolers' attachment classifications: *The circle of security intervention. Journal of Consulting and Clinical Psychology, 74*(6), 1017–1026. https://doi.org/10.1037/0022-006X.74.6.1017
9. Ginsburg, K. R. (2007). The importance of play in promoting healthy child development and maintaining strong parent-child bonds. *Pediatrics, 119,* 182–191.
10. Chazan, S. E. (2002). *Profiles of play: Assessing and observing structure and process in play therapy.* Jessica Kingsley Publishers.
11. Raising Kids Network. (2022). Retrieved from https://raisingchildren.net.au/preschoolers/play-learning/active-play/rough-play-guide
12. Locatelli, M. G. (2020). Play therapy treatment of pediatric medical trauma: A retrospective case study of a preschool child. *International Journal of Play Therapy, 29*(1), 33–42. https://doi.org/10.1037/pla0000109

Therapeutic Play and Aiding Purpose in the Preschooler

Leanne Hallowell

Objectives

At the end of this chapter, you will be able to:

- Develop an understanding of Erikson's psychosocial development stage of initiative verses guilt and how this may be impacted when children are hospitalised.
- Identify how therapeutic play may minimise the impact of hospitalisation and aid purpose in the preschooler.
- Identify how relationships between parents and health care professionals and developmentally sensitive communication can support the reduction of anxiety, whilst supporting the development of resilience and coping in children.

Introduction

This chapter focuses on caring for preschool children aged between 3 and 5 years. It considers child development and assessment and incorporates Erikson's psychosocial developmental stage of initiative versus guilt. Considerations for nursing and allied health care and the integration of therapeutic play approaches to support young children, siblings and their parents as partners are included.

Play is critical for the healthy development of children. Play provides space for physical, emotional, cognitive, and social development. Obstacles which may impede or negatively impact play and developmental progression include hospitalisation and potentially painful medical procedures. Children between 3 and 5 years of age, preschoolers, are noted by Erikson [1] to be in the third stage of development, 'initiative versus guilt' and are beginning to assert power and control over

L. Hallowell (✉)
Faculty of Education and Arts, Australian Catholic University (ACU),
Melbourne, VIC, Australia

© The Author(s), under exclusive license to Springer Nature
Switzerland AG 2022
J. A. Parson et al. (eds.), *Integrating Therapeutic Play Into Nursing and Allied Health Practice*, https://doi.org/10.1007/978-3-031-16938-0_8

their world through the direction of their play and social interactions. Successful completion of this stage of development leads to a sense of initiative and the virtue of purpose. The helplessness that can come with hospitalisation and medical procedures may result in a child not achieving the initiative required to successfully accomplish milestones in the preschool stage of psychosocial development.

Although the need for play increases when a child is hospitalised, play in hospital may in fact be suppressed [2]. The suppression of play may be due to the child's medical condition and a diminished ability or desire to play; reduced opportunity for play due to limited resources, space, or the child not having actual or perceived permission to play. The integration of play and playful approaches (including in a playroom, isolation room, or in a hospital bed) may provide children with a sense of initiative and can be used to support children to engage in impending medical procedures. Parents can also be involved throughout hospitalisation and engaged in medical procedures. When parents and siblings are involved, the child feels a sense of normality and continuation, providing a sense of security. Further, Graves and Larkins [3] note when parents encourage, support, and communicate with their child, showing understanding and tolerance, they support the building of confidence and resilience.

Child Development and Assessment

Children reach developmental milestones at different rates. However, when hospitalised, there may be some regression which a typically developing child will regain. However, engaging children in play whilst in hospital, whilst building confidence and resilience is also known to minimise regression [4]. Assessing children prior to hospitalisation in relation to their physical, social, emotional, cognitive, and language development is critical to support discussions regarding care, and planning playful interventions related to impending hospitalisation and medical procedures. This allows interventions to be planned to meet the specific needs of the child and their family.

Physical Development

In terms of gross motor skills, healthy children, 3–5 years of age, can dress and undress with little help, they can catch and throw balls, and climb playground equipment. Their fine motor skills are also developing. Hand preference is noted, as is an ability to imitate shapes when drawing and cutting with scissors. Assessing this in a medical context may be undertaken as part of the medical assessment. Questions may be directed at the child, 'Do you like to throw a ball? Can you throw a ball with one hand or two?' The child may even be engaged in a game of catch, making the medical assessment fun [5]. This can also be assessed through observation by allowing the child access to drawing implements or asking if they can remove parts of their clothing during a medical assessment. If a child is experiencing illness or injury, their physical capabilities may be impacted, and this will need to be considered when determining what part of their medical treatment a child has the physical capacity to assist with.

Psychosocial Development

Play provides a context for the child to continue their usual activities [2] and a space for communication and self-expression [6]. Bruner [7] notes that play minimises the consequence of one's actions and of learning, and that it provides an 'opportunity to try out combinations of behaviour that would under functional pressure, never be tried' (p.693).

Socialisation skills are developed in play [8]. Associative play and cooperative play are distinct forms of play seen in children from 3 years of age. Associative play occurs as children begin to play together. When children engage in more sophisticated cooperative play, typically from around four and a half years, they begin to negotiate with others. Social development at this age can be observed by engaging in conversation with the child, keeping in mind the age of the child and their developing language abilities. Questions such as 'How many friends do you have at kindergarten? What is your best friend? What do you like to do when you play with them?' may elicit an understanding of the child's social world. It is expected that a child aged 3–5 years will enjoy playing with others and may have a particular friend. Alternatively, the child could be provided with play-based activities such as drawing a picture or showing with toys how they play with their friends. These types of show and tell activities rely less on verbal language ability and allow the child to communicate through the language of play.

Erikson [1] suggests that at this 'play age' the child understands and comforts another, but also responds to affection and praise—given and received. This suggests that as health care professionals engage with children in this context, there needs to be a focus on exploring the strengths children exhibit, such as what the child does well prior to a medical intervention, throughout the intervention, and to unpack positives post intervention. It is acknowledged that concerns and fears may be evident in relation to a procedure, however, in the lead up to and throughout a medical procedure itself, to maximise coping, refine self-regulation skills, and to minimise pain, the focus needs to be on the child's strengths and abilities [9]. A child's attachment with the caregiver is also vital at this stage of development. Attachment theory notes the need for a committed caregiving relationship with at least one adult fig [10]. and a secure base from which to explore [11]. In supporting a child through hospitalisation and medical procedures, Karlsson et al. [12] observe that the attachment relationship can be tested. Children typically want parents to be present during medical procedures [13] and they should be encouraged by nursing and allied health staff to use supportive measures, such as play and talk, to meet their child's needs. In supporting their child through distraction and/or nonprocedural talk, parents are in fact protecting their child and providing a 'secure base'.

Language Development

Children aged 3–5 years, in the initiative versus guilt stage, can and do speak in sentences, ask questions (many questions), and can answer questions. Typically, they can take part in conversation, and enjoy experimenting with new words. Rather than seeing questions as trivial or a nuisance, they should be understood to reflect a child's current need to understand and should be responded to with care and consideration. Hospitalisations and medical procedures can provide children with many new words. However, it is critical that the practitioner does not assume that a child understands these words. When providing a child with a medical term, defining the term can provide context and reduce confusion and anxiety. Explaining that 'a small tube will be left in your arm so we can give you medicine when we need to. We will take the small tube out when you don't need the medicine anymore', is more easily understood by a young child, than 'we need to cannulate you'.

Understanding a child's ability to take on new knowledge helps the health care professional to pitch the language they use about impending medical procedures in a way the child can understand. Knowing if a child understands positional words, not limited to big and little, and middle and end, can follow simple instructions and provide simple answers and recall events, provides health practitioners with an understanding of the child's capacity to understand words that may be used to describe medical procedures and to adapt their explanation to the child. When a child does not have a context for a word or concept, they will replace it with something they do understand. For example, the author asked a child if they could tell her why they were at the hospital. The child told the author that they were there to have a 'scan'. When asked if he could tell the author about the scan, the child answered that he could not tell her, but he could draw it. When the child spoke about the drawing, he described a handheld scanner used in grocery stores. This was his known context. Although he was able to recall the event correctly, expected as part of this stage of cognitive development, it was a transference of his knowledge, in this case a single word, into a different context which created confusion for the child that needed to be unpacked with the help of a health care professional. Piaget [14] referred to this as assimilation. The child understood what a scan was, however, additional information expanded and developed his knowledge of a scan in a medical context.

Neurological Development

Neurological development is at its greatest before a child reaches the age of 5 years. At this age the brain of a child has developed by 90% [15]. In the period between 2–7 years of age, further myelination and development of dendrites occurs in the brain's cortex. The left hemisphere, typically involved with language skills, grows dramatically. The right hemisphere, which grows throughout childhood, is involved in tasks which require spatial skills. As this occurs there is a corresponding change in the child's capabilities. As well as the development of thinking, children are better able to strategise, and control attention and emotion [16], and the child is increasingly able to understand their environment. However, in unusual circumstances, such as being hospitalised or requiring medical intervention, children will need additional support to feel safe and make sense of this unfamiliar environment.

Play Development

'Play is a context for learning that allows for the expression of personality and uniqueness; enhances dispositions such as curiosity and creativity; enables children to make connections between prior experiences and new learning; assists children to develop relationships and concepts; stimulates a sense of wellbeing' ([17], p 10). Although play is easily recognised when observed, play has no formal or agreed definition. Typically play has broad and general definitions and elements of play can be found in, but are not limited to, games, sports, language, competitions, and art. Whilst play may appear to have no intended serious purpose, play is important for physical, social, emotional, and cognitive development [18]. Jean Piaget [19] theorised that the make-believe play of young children provides them with opportunities to play out real-life conflicts and to discover and work through possible resolutions. Sutton-Smith [20] suggests that play can be used as an expression of frustration, to cope with and manage environmental challenges. Erikson [1] proposed that play allows children opportunities to experiment with a range of experiences and to consider possible real-life consequences, in safe settings.

In a medical setting, play can help reduce a child's anxiety and concerns related to their health condition or hospitalisation [21]. Being able to play imaginatively can be an adaptive coping mechanism that aids mastery over challenging experiences and provides stress inoculation [22, 23]. Stress inoculation may also include play-based activities that encourage muscle relaxation, breathing exercises, cognitive restructuring, and guided imagery. Play can also illicit information about the child's knowledge of their medical condition or treatment. The health care professional may engage children in art or play-based activities. For example, asking the child, 'could you draw me a picture of the machine that will take pictures of your sore arm', or 'can you draw on this doll where you are feeling sore' will give the health care professional useful knowledge and insight into the child's view of their medical care.

Considerations for Nursing and Allied Health

Preschool children are at what Piaget referred to as the preoperational stage of cognitive development [14]. When children are at this stage of development, provision of procedural information should include the use of appropriate resources such as images, (still or moving), and/or medical props. The use of concrete resources can provide clarity to new knowledge. Children who have been supported in this way have opportunities to accommodate this new knowledge and will report lower levels of anxiety and pain. Further, this will support prevention of negative distortions or exaggerations in the later recall of events. Noel et al. [24] found that children who reported high levels of pain immediately following a medical procedure tended to overestimate this level over time whilst children who had been exposed to distraction and coping behaviours were more likely to accurately recall details of the procedure.

In terms of the provision of new knowledge, this is most effective for children in the preoperational stage if the focus is on external, concrete events. This may involve the provision of procedural descriptions, such as what will take place and where, as well as sensory descriptions, such as what they might feel, hear, or smell [25]. For example, part of the work of the author was to support children to develop strategies for the induction of anaesthesia. A variety of tools were used, including images of the room where the induction would take place, explanations of what the equipment was and what and how it was used in this process (and what would not be used), and opportunities to practise the use of a mask for the provision of anaesthetic gases (often on a doll first). In this process, children were provided with information about the temperature of the induction room and asked if they wanted a blanket to keep warm. They could also change the smell of the mask—essence was wiped on the inside of the mask to alter the smell to one of their choosing. Supporting children to be agentic in how processes are managed further develops coping mechanisms.

Being hospitalised, pain, fatigue, social isolation, and treatment regimens are likely to compromise the play of hospitalised children [26]. Adaptive capacities and the resilience of children are impacted when unable to participate in playful activities. Typically, health care professionals focus on the biological facets of treatment and are less inclined to address social and emotional facets. Nijhof and colleagues note that there is a relationship between stress, play, and resilience in children [26]. Children who are stressed or anxious are less likely to engage in playful behaviour [27] whilst children themselves report that play is one of the coping strategies that they are most likely to use [13]. Shields [28] noted that feeling a lack of control may increase in children who are hospitalised, with daily routines interrupted, an unfamiliar environment, and with strange and unfamiliar medical procedures. Children may behave in ways which suggest defiance as they try to navigate this new environment. Opportunities that allow the child to show initiative, to be in control, to make choices when appropriate, and to use coping strategies where they are actively involved, are vital through all aspects of the hospital journey.

Common Fears and Anxieties

Hospitalisation is rarely a choice children make. What is important for children of this age is to explain why hospitalisation needs to occur and to offer choices that are realistic for the child. An explanation of why a child needs to go to hospital should be clear, developmentally sensitive, and provide opportunities for the child and family to ask questions and seek clarification. Lerwick (2017) notes that hospitalised children can be subject to psychological trauma, which may manifest as anxiety, aggression, and anger. Hospitalised children also lack control over their environment and this sense of helplessness, coupled with fear and pain, may cause children to feel powerless. Children may fear mutilation, and suffer from guilt, pain, or rage [13], often because processes are ill-explained or their voices not heard [29]. Often the most significant fear for a child and their family is that of the unknown. Explanations to the child and their family may include what has happened or is happening to their body and an explanation of what the treatment options may be. This needs to be undertaken in a way that is developmentally appropriate for the child. By involving the family, the fears and anxieties of the family are also minimised. When children feel helpless and out of control, the cooperation which is required for the smooth undertaking of medical procedures and treatment may be lost. Choice empowers the child. Children will feel more in control when they know what to expect [30].

Grief and Loss

Children may feel bewildered in an unknown medical environment, and as medical and allied health staff take control over their bodies, they may feel a loss of autonomy and control. Further, this sense of loss can be heightened if they feel their body is failing them. Pain or changes in mobility are examples of this. Heightened by potential misunderstandings of what is happening or about to happen, children of this age do not have the ability to understand the complexities of their experience and will consider things from their developmental viewpoint. For example, they may think that all the equipment in the room will be used on them when in fact it may not, or being put to sleep, meaning they will not wake up from an operation. Stanford [31] outlines language considerations when talking about pain and procedures with children. He noted that words with dual meanings should be avoided, 'put to sleep' being one. Children who have heard the word 'sleep' in the context of explaining a death may misconstrue its meaning in a medical context.

Pain Management

Potentially painful procedures can be supported in several ways to minimise the chance of a child experiencing medical trauma. Children need to be reassured that there are things they can do, along with their parents and the medical staff to help minimise the pain and discomfort they may feel during a procedure. It is also important that health care professionals are honest in their explanations. Rather than responding to a child that they will not feel pain, statements such as 'some children say it hurts a bit, others are not so bothered' is a more honest approach. This would be followed by reassurance that there are things that can be done to make it easier such as medication, distraction techniques, and controlled breathing exercises.

Explanations about the procedure should include a description of why the procedure needs to occur and how it will help them, what happens in the procedure, where it will happen, and what the child might feel. The timing of the explanation is important. Timing the provision of new knowledge will influence how readily a child is able to attend to, process and act on the new knowledge [25]. Generally, for children aged 3–5 years, in the preoperational stage, this should be in the lead up, not immediately (if it can be avoided) before the procedure happens. Limited new information should be provided just before and/or during the procedure. Once a procedure is underway, the child will then benefit from assistance in applying coping strategies. Providing information about medical procedures too early can increase a child's anticipatory anxiety [32]. Furthermore, children will retain very little information a week after being told (Eiser & Patterson, 1983). If information is provided too close to a medical procedure, a child will have limited time to process the information or to develop coping strategies [33]. Ideally children should be provided with information 1 or 2 days prior to the procedure. Decisions around timing the provision of new knowledge may be further impacted by the child's temperament and coping style and the type of admission. In terms of emergency admissions, there may not be the option to consider timing the provision of new knowledge.

Providing choice as to how a procedure may be carried out can also be empowering. For example, a child may be provided with options regarding what position a procedure may occur in, for example, they may be able to sit or lie on a parent's lap, hug their parent, or provided with a choice regarding the site of the cannula. Other choices could include deciding which clothes/nightwear to pack or allowing the child to take off their own clothes during a medical exam and only those which need to be removed. Doing this in a way that is sensitive to the need for privacy. Choice can also be as simple as asking, 'I need to listen to your heart and to look in your ears, which shall I do first?' In doing this, it is noted that this needs to happen, the choice is in which order. Furthermore, adding why each needs to be done supports knowledge development. Small shifts in language can foster empowerment, and the development of an environment of trust and safety.

Further intervention after the procedure can also provide comfort. For children aged 3–5 years, it can be helpful to discuss what they did well, as this optimises their memory, that is their recall is enhanced and distress is reduced [34]. This will have positive implications for future medical procedures. There will always be something positive you can mention to provide a sense of achievement which can support a child to return for a further procedure if required. When 'bookended' with positive experiences before and after a medical procedure, negative associations can be reduced, and positive associations become the starting point for future medical interventions [35].

Therapeutic Play Approaches for Clinical Practice

A key application of therapeutic play approaches for the preschool child is the use of distraction techniques during medical procedures. It is important that suitable distraction techniques are developed with the children and their family so that everyone has 'their own job' to focus on. The types of distraction used will be based on the child's interests, capabilities, and choice. Distraction techniques may include 'blowing away scary feelings or any hurt', blowing bubbles or a windmill, counting games, using a search and find book (also useful as a visual block), and mind pictures (where the child describes a picture in their mind and responds to questions about it). Counting games can be as simple as counting bubbles, or how many lights are on the ceiling. Search and find books, can also be used as a tool for counting. Holding the book between the site of the cannulation or procedure and the child, creates a visual block and keeps the focus on the book as a distraction tool. It is important that the child knows that whilst they are counting or looking for items in the book, the procedure will continue.

Parents as Partners

The impact of hospitalisation is not limited to the child themselves, but extends to the entire family [36]. In any intervention to prepare children for medical procedures, families, where possible, should be included. Families also need support in understanding what may happen to the child, how the child may be feeling, and what they may understand. Families can also be provided with strategies to support their child, including creating opportunities for the child to engage in physical and imaginative play, and supporting the child to make choices within safe boundaries. Giving children the freedom to make appropriate choices and to engage in play reinforces a sense of initiative. When health care providers identify and work with the strengths of children and their parents, they support the establishment of a trusting relationship. Space should be provided to normalise common fears and anxiety, and for the child and their family to have their feelings and perspectives recognised. Vasey et al. [44] found that parents want to be involved in their child's care and in supporting the management of pain. Furthermore, parental involvement in medical procedures is known to improve the child's overall experience, reduce anxiety and improve satisfaction in care [37].

Chapter Summary

Within the health care setting children need information/new knowledge provided in a way that is age appropriate, developmentally sensitive, and tailored specifically to their needs. Furthermore, children need opportunities to engage in suitable play activities to minimise the impact of hospitalisations and potential painful procedures, relieve anxiety, assist them to make sense of medical procedures, and support the development of resilience. Key to this is the relationship between parents and the health care professional, so that sensitive communication occurs to support development and coping in children within the medical setting.

Reflective Questions and Activities

- A key element to providing new knowledge about impending medical procedures and hospitalisation to young children is to engage in conversations that will
elicit information about what they already know. Consider a series of questions
or playful activities you could use with a young child to unearth this information.
- In discussion with a child and their family, you discover that a previous medical
procedure had been stressful. Develop a plan for how you would address this to
support better outcomes for the child and family prior to the next medical
procedure.

References

1. Erikson, E. H. (1977). *Toys and reason: Stages in the ritualisation of experience.* W.W. Norton Company.
2. Koukourikos, K., Tzeha, L., Pantelidou, P., & Tsalogidou, A. (2015). The importance of play during hospitalisation of children. Materia socio-Medica. *The Journal of Academy of Medical Sciences of Bosnia and Herzegovina, 6*, 438–441. https://doi.org/10.5455/msm.2015.27.438-441
3. Graves, S. B., & Larkin, E. (2006). Lessons from Erikson. A look at autonomy across the lifespan. *Journal of Intergenerational Relationships, 4*(2), 61–71. https://doi.org/10.1300/J194v04n02_05
4. Caplin, D., & Cooper, M. (2007). Child development in inpatient medicine. In L. B. Zaoutis & V. W. Chiang (Eds.), *Comprehensive pediatric hospital medicine, (pp.1285–1292).* Elsevier. https://doi.org/10.1016/B978-032303004-5.50219-2
5. Alexander, K., & Mazza, D. (2010). How to perform a 'healthy kids check'. *Australian Family Physician, 39*(10), 760–765.
6. Dell Clark, C. (2003). *In sickness and in play: Children coping with chronic illness.* University Press.
7. Bruner, J. S. (1972). Nature and uses of immaturity. *American Psychologist, 27*(8), 687–708. https://doi.org/10.1037/h0033144
8. Parten, M. B. (1933). Social play among preschool children. *The Journal of Abnormal and Social Psychology, 28*(2), 136–147. https://doi.org/10.1037/h0073939
9. Kohen, D. P., & Kaiser, P. (2014). Clinical hypnosis with children and adolescents, what? Why? How?: Origins, applications and efficacy. *Children, 1*, 74–98. https://doi.org/10.3390/children1020074
10. Bretherton, I. (1992). The origins of attachment theory. John Bowlby and Mary Ainsworth. *Developmental Psychology, 28*, 759–775.
11. Ainsworth, M. D. S. (1963). The development of mother-infant interaction among the Ganda. In B. M. Foss (Ed.), *Determinants of infant behaviour* (pp. 67–104). Wiley.
12. Karlsson, K., Englund, A. C., Enskar, K., & Rydstrom, I. (2014). Parents perspectives in supporting children during needle-related medical procedures. *International Journal of Qualitative Studies on Health and Well-Being, 9*(1). https://doi.org/10.3401/qw.v9.23759
13. Salmela, M., Salantera, S., Ruotsalainen, T., & Aronen, E. T. (2010). Coping strategies for hospital-related fears in pre-school-aged children. *Journal of Pediatric Child Health, 46*(3), 108–114. https://doi.org/10.1111/j.1440-1754.2009.01647.x
14. Piaget, J. (1952). *The Origins of Intelligence in children.* (M.Cook, Trans). W.W. Norton you & Co. https://doi.org/10.1037/11494-000
15. Brown, T. T., & Jernigan, T. L. (2012). Brain development during the preschool years. *Neuropsychology Review, 22*, 313–333. https://doi.org/10.1007/s11065-012-9214-1

16. Halfon, N., Shulman, E., & Shulman, M. (2001). Brain development in early childhood. Building community for young children. (reports - descriptive 141). UCLA Center for healthier children. *Families and Communities.*

17. Department of Education and Training. (2019, March 6). Belonging *The Early Years Learning Framework for Australia.* Department of Education, Skills and Employment retrieved March 26, 2022.

18. Bateson, P. (2015). Playfulness and creativity. *Current Biology, 25,* R12–R16.

19. Piaget, J. (1962). *Play, dreams and imitation in childhood.* W.W. Norton & Company.

20. Sutton-Smith, B. (2008). Play theory - a personal journey of new thoughts. *American Journal of Play, 2008*(1), 80–123.

21. Li, W. H. C., Chung, J. O. K., Ho, K. Y., & Kwok, B. M. C. (2016). Play interventions to reduce anxiety and negative emotions in hospitalised children. *BMC Pediatrics, 16*(36). https://doi.org/10.1186/s12887-016-0570-5

22. Cavett, A. M. (2013). In S. Inoculation, I. C. J. Schaefer, & A. A. Drews (Eds.), *The therapeutic powers of play. 20 Core agents of change* (pp. 132–141). John Wiley & Sons.

23. Jay, S. M., & Elliott, C. H. (1990). A stress inoculation program for parents whose children are undergoing painful medical procedures. *Journal of Consulting and Clinical Psychology, 58*(6), 799–804. https://doi.org/10.1037/0022-006X.58.6.799

24. Noel, M., McMurtry, C. M., Chambers, C. T., & McGrath, P. J. (2010). Children's memory for painful procedures: The relationship of pain intensity, anxiety and adult behaviours to subsequent recall. *Journal of Pediatric Psychology., 35*(6), 626–636. https://doi.org/10.1093/jpepsy/jsp096

25. Janniste, T., Hayes, B., & von Baeyer, C. L. (2004). Providing children with information about medical procedures.: A review and synthesis. *Clinical Psychology: Science and Practice, 14*(2), 124–143.

26. Niijhof, S. L., Vinkers, C. H., van Geelen, S. M., Duijff, S. N., Achterberg, E. J. M., van der Net, J., Veltkamp, R. C., Grootenhuis, M. A., van de Putte, E. M., Hillegers, M. H. J., van der Burg, A. W., Wierenga, C. J., Benders, M. J. N. L., Engles, R. C. M. E., van der Ent, K., Vanderschuren, J. M. J., & Lesscher, H. M. B. (2018). Healthy play, better coping: The importance of play for the development of children in health and disease. *Neuroscience and Biobehavioural Reviews, 95,* 421–429.

27. Castelhano, A. S., Scorza, F. A., Teixeira, M. C., Arida, R. M., Cavalheiro, E. A., & Cysneiros, R. M. (2010). Social play impairment following status epileptics during early development. *Journal of Neural Transmission, 117*(10), 1155–1160.

28. Shields, L. (2001). A review of the literature from developed and developing countries relating to the effects of hospitalisation on children and parents. *International Nursing Review., 28*(10), 29–37.

29. United Nations Convention on the Rights of the Child, November 20, 1989, Retrieved April 24, 2022, from https://www.ohchr.org/en/professionalinterest/pages/crc.aspx

30. Hockenberry, M. J., & Wilson, D. (2014). *Wong's.* Nursing Care of Infants and Children.

31. Stanford, G. (1991). Beyond honesty: Choosing language for asking children about pain and procedures. *Children's Health Care, 20*(4), 261–262. https://doi.org/10.1207/s15326888chc2004_11

32. Melamed, B. G., & Ridley-Johnson, R. (1988). Psychological preparation of families for hospitalization. *Journal of Developmental and Behavioural Pediatrics, 9*(2), 96–102.

33. Kain, Z. N., Mayes, L. C., & Caramico, L. A. (1996). Preoperative preparation in children: A cross-sectional study. *Journal of Clinical Anesthesia, 8*(6), 508–514. https://doi.org/10.1016/0952-8180(96)00115-8

34. Salmon, K., McGuigan, F., & Pereira, J. K. (2006). Brief report: Optimising children's memory and management of an invasive medical procedure: The influence of procedural narration and distraction. *Journal of Pediatric Psychology, 31*(5), 522–527.

35. Cini, C. (2020). Royal Childrens Hospital: Clinical Procedure Pain Management Guideline. Retrieved April 21, 2022, from https://www.rch.org.au/rchcpg/hospital_clinical_guideline_index/Procedure_Management_Guideline/#After

36. Christin, A., Akre, C., Berchtold, A., & Suris, J. C. (2016). Parent-adolescent relationship in youths with a chronic condition. *Child: Care, Health and Development, 42*(1), 36–41.
37. Vasey, J., Smith, J., Kirschbaum, M. N., & Chirema, K. (2018). Tokenism or true partnership: Parental involvement in a child's acute pain. *Journal of Clinical Nursing, 28*, 1491–1505. https://doi.org/10.1111/jocn.14

Therapeutic Play and Instilling Competence in the School-Aged Child

Sarah Hickson

Chapter Objectives

At the end of this chapter, you will be able to:

- Demonstrate a basic understanding of the key milestones associated with the development of school-aged children 5–13 years.
- Describe Erikson's fourth stage of psychosocial development, industry verse inferiority, and how this applies to the school-aged child.
- Consider the use of therapeutic play techniques to engage the school-aged child in a developmentally sensitive manner in the health care setting.

Introduction

The school-age years are an important stage of development where a child's social world expands. Understanding how children present based on typical developmental expectations is essential knowledge for health care practitioners. This chapter will focus on school-aged children 5–13 years. Incorporating Erikson's fourth stage of psychosocial development, industry verse inferiority, the chapter will explore several key elements that contribute to healthy development and instilling competence in the school-aged child. The use of therapeutic play techniques within the health care setting will also be explored.

S. Hickson (✉)
Private Practice, London, UK

J. A. Parson et al. (eds.), *Integrating Therapeutic Play Into Nursing and Allied Health Practice*, https://doi.org/10.1007/978-3-031-16938-0_9

Child Development and Assessment

Physical Development

Children reach many physical milestones during the school years as their understanding of themselves and the world around them develops. It is important to acknowledge that some children may progress at a different rate than others depending on individual circumstances, including genetics, environmental factors and early childhood experiences. Some of the common physical milestones children may reach at this stage include the ability to distinguish between their left and right, independence in self-care tasks such as bathing and dressing, the ability to ride a bicycle, jump, skip and chase, as well as an increased ability to use tools, such as eating utensils [1]. Children of school age need plenty of opportunities for physical activity to assist in building strength, coordination and confidence in themselves and their physical abilities. Physical activity can also enhance a child's academic performance, increase their self-esteem and prevent obesity and serious illnesses in the future, such as diabetes [2].

During this stage of development, children will have an increased body awareness which may lead to an increase in physical complaints, which may be related to their physical development, illness or injury. Regardless of the nature of a physical complaint, it should not be dismissed, so that any underlying health condition or emotional concerns can be explored. For children who have experienced significant trauma, it is not uncommon for these children to complain of physical ailments. Whilst these complaints may not have a physical cause they may reflect an unmet emotional need. No matter how small or big, health care professionals should always check and tend to these 'hurts' giving the message that 'you are important, I want to help you with your hurts, and I care about you'.

Psychosocial Development

Developmental psychologists have theorised about the psychosocial processes involved in development. Psychologist Jean Piaget identified four stages of cognitive development. Piaget's theory explains how the child not only acquires knowledge as they develop but also create a mental model of the world [3]. During the school years, a child is said to be at the *Concrete Operational Stage*. During this stage, children become less egocentric and begin to understand that not everyone shares their thoughts, beliefs or feelings [4]. Piaget believed that a child's cognitive development was dependent on changes in a child's cognitive processing ability. Piaget observed that children learn and develop in sequence. However, Piaget's theory did not extend to the child in relation to their social context, which in the school years, becomes significant. Alternatively, Lev Vygotsky focused on a child's community and believed that it held a critical role in how children learn to make sense of the world. He believed that a child's observations and experiences of the community around them will make meaning out of everything they see, learn, feel and hear [5]. Unlike other developmental psychologists, Erikson not only examined child development but the whole human lifespan, from birth to death [6]. The school-age years are known as Erikson's fourth stage of psychosocial development, industry verse inferiority. Successful resolution of the crisis that accompanies this stage of development results in the virtue of competence. The developmental stages before the school years focus on the influence of caregivers and family members. From the school years the focus widens to include the greater social network around the child, including peers. These new social interactions influence a child's confidence, self-esteem and self-concept.

By the school-age years, children can understand emotions in a more complex way. They understand that someone else can feel differently and be able to operate recursively on this understanding [7]. At this age, children are also more likely to make comparisons between themselves and others. A child observing their peers completing tasks may discover that they are more or less able than their peers. This experience is likely to influence how the child perceives themselves in relation to others. In other words, the child may increase in confidence and self-esteem if they experience a sense of achievement compared to another child, especially if their abilities receive praise and validation from others. Here they gain a sense of industry—they feel competent in their ability. However, a child may decrease in confidence and experience feelings of inadequacy and low self-esteem if they feel their abilities are less than those of their peers, here they may experience feelings of inferiority.

A child's early attachment experiences also impact on the development of a child's sense of competence. A child's strategy of attachment will influence how the child responds in relationships. Bowlby [8] believed that if a child experiences a secure attachment with a caregiver, they take this security with them into the tasks of life. They are less dependent on external validation, less devastated by failure and less in need of status to reassure themselves of their own worth. These children carry with them a stable, measured and secure sense of who they are. When it comes to the school-aged child these early attachment experiences will shape a child's ability to regulate their level of emotional arousal. A school-aged child who has experienced a complex and emotionally challenging environment with an unavailable or unpredictable caregiver is likely to respond differently to a child who has experienced an available and consistent caregiver. If the stages before act as a blueprint for what is to come next in relation to the self and others, children with difficult attachment experiences may also have difficulty forming positive peer relationships which may impact on their capacity to develop a sense of industry at this stage of development. Children who have difficulty interacting with peers are at risk for social difficulties [9]. Some of these difficulties may include an inability to recognise emotions in oneself and others, respond appropriately and communicate effectively. This may then lead to future problems with mental health, maintaining friendships or low academic performance. A child's eligibility for play and group activities enables them to meet their social needs and provides opportunities for genuine personality development and the creation of healthy peer relationships [10].

Neurological Development

Two important brain growth spurts occur during the school-age years [11]. Between the age of 6 and 8 years, there are significant improvements in fine motor skills and eye–hand coordination. A second growth spurt occurs between 10 and 12 years, where the frontal lobes become more developed leading to an increased capacity for logic, planning and memory (Molen & Molenaar 1994). School-age children are also better able to plan and coordinate activity using both left and right hemispheres of the brain, and to control emotional outbursts. Attention is also improved as the prefrontal cortex matures [12].

During this stage the emotional brain also develops considerably. Siegel [13] explores the link between social interactions and how the mind develops meaning. He describes how meaning making and relationships appear to be mediated via the same neural circuits responsible for initiating emotional processes. Emotion can therefore be seen as an integrating process that links the internal and interpersonal worlds of the human mind [13]. Essentially at this stage, the brain is molded by learning and social influences. It is an optimal time for learning because children are developing critical and abstract thinking skills. They are becoming more skilled in reading, writing and linguistics [14]. In play, they may now be able to create their own games with complicated rules. At this age, children need opportunities to practice and repeat skills such as bike riding, swimming and cleaning their teeth.

Trauma, abuse or neglect can have a negative impact on the developing brain. These changes can have lifelong physical and psychological consequences. Perry [15] observes the brain's sensitivity to adverse experiences in early childhood and how this has the potential to impact on brain development and emotional, behavioural, cognitive, social and physiological functioning.

Play Development

The power of play is incredibly profound and is crucial to a child's development. Frequently in the school-age years, there is an emphasis on intellectual development which can overshadow social and emotional development. Play can allow children to freely express themselves, it is not dependent on how well a child is doing in science or how skilled they are at remembering mathematical equations. Play not only aids the development of the self but also the development of relationships with others. For example, children can learn about turn taking through games with simple rules. Learning how to play fairly and equally can help a child develop skills in making and maintaining friendships. Games with rules and simple structures can also help a child to develop skills that assist them in managing timetables and learning frameworks at school. According to Vygotsky [16], efficient learning occurs in a social context, where learning is scaffolded into meaningful contexts that resonate with children's active engagement and previous experiences. Children learn through the enjoyment of the play and increase their confidence, self-worth and sense of industry through the achievements they experience whilst playing. Older children tend to become increasingly interested in play involving risk and challenge. For example, a child might want to ride their bike down a steep hill or reach the highest point of the climbing frame in the playground. As well as learning about their physical limits, they are developing their problem-solving skills as they negotiate risk through play.

Jennings [17] has developed two interweaving developmental paradigms for play, Neuro-Dramatic-Play (NDP) and Embodiment-Projection-Role (EPR). NDP begins in infancy and continues until 6 months, whilst EPR follows the progression of dramatic play from birth to 7 years. By the school-age years, the child is in the 'role stage'. The child's play becomes increasingly dramatised including stories and scenes being enacted. At this stage, children build confidence and increase skills in communication through being able to play roles in superhero and fantasy stories, improvise with new ideas to set a scene and create masks and costumes to develop characters. EPR addresses the physical, cognitive, emotional and social developmental stages of the young child. Children can experience EPR through play, dance, games, singing, movement, stories and sensory experiences. With myths and fairy tales, the child can experience different roles and identities, relationships as well as explore risk and resolution. Jennings [18] suggests that competence in NDP and EPR are essential to maturity due to their influence on early attachment, formation of emotional intelligence, problem solving and conflict resolution. In the school-age child, role play will also contribute to the development of the skills needed to navigate the social world.

Through play, school-aged children can feel competent and gain a sense of industry. Everyday play is not scored or graded. For the school-aged child, it can also help children escape the pressure and focus on academic achievement. An overemphasis on academic learning may lead a child to constantly compare themselves to their peers. There is a risk for school-age children to feel inferior when the focus weighs heavily on academic progression. Every child can be successful and feel competent at something if given the right opportunity. Broadening the horizon of what these opportunities look like can give every child a chance to experience a sense of industry. Play can offer every child a place to grow, learn, achieve and feel good about something.

Considerations for Nursing and Allied Health Care

Common Fears and Anxieties

Young school children are likely to feel afraid and anxious when engaging with services including health and therapeutic care. At this stage of self and social awareness, they may be worried about what is the matter with them or nervous about interacting with strange professionals. Children will often use behaviour to communicate how they feel, especially in situations of stress and uncertainty. A child may become aggressive or withdrawn. This may become problematic for assessment or medical procedures, so it is essential that appropriate therapeutic skills are applied to help create a safe space and foundation of trust for the child. For a particularly nervous child, allowing time for the child to relax into the appointment is important. They will need the support of their parent/caregiver and preparation for what to expect. As well as a nurturing and inviting physical environment. Building rapport and developing trust with the child will help ease anxieties and lessen the child's fear and anxiety.

Grief and Loss/Death and Dying

Children have an awareness of death from a relatively young age, although they may not fully understand it. Children of school age have the capacity to understand the permanence of death [19]. It is therefore important they are provided with the facts in an age-appropriate way using developmentally sensitive language. A sensitive approach is needed to avoid overwhelming children with too much information that may scare or confuse them. Overly complicated terms and details may be hard for a child to understand. Not enough explanation, however, such as saying a person has 'gone to sleep', may lead to confusion and the false belief that the person is going to wake up again. It is best to listen and answer any questions that may arise sensitively and honestly, no matter how big or small.

However, loss does not always mean death and can refer to losses including the loss of a parent through severed relationships such as divorce, the loss of friendships in schools, the loss of a favourite teacher or the loss of an ability due to illness or injury. No matter what the loss is, grieving for that loss is important. Children grieve and cope differently than adults. They are likely to act out how they are feeling through their behaviour rather than verbalise it. They may become withdrawn or emotionally reactive. Although expressed differently, children still experience powerful feelings, so it is important their experiences are not minimised. Support needs to be developmentally appropriate. Children of school age need to be encouraged to grieve and be able to express their feelings both verbally and non-verbally through play, art and creativity. Children's books about death, such as Badgers Parting Gifts by Susan Varley, can be read with a trusted adult to help start conversations about loss. We know how important play is at any stage of child development, especially when words are just too hard. Drawing pictures and telling stories are examples of the many ways to help a child express a feeling of loss.

Pain Management

When a child of school age is in pain, they may not always verbally communicate this. Some behaviours that may indicate distress include a loss of appetite, insomnia, crying, lack of play, increased sedentary behaviour, irritability and physical sensitivity. Therefore, observing how a child is behaving is as important as listening to what they are saying. Children will need comfort in times of pain through the presence of a caregiver. A transitional object may also provide comfort. The concept of a transitional object was introduced by Winnicott [20]. A transitional object is something which represents the mother–child bond. Common examples include soft toys, dolls or blankets. By having a familiar object, the child may feel a sense of psychological comfort and security in anxious times, such as when receiving medical care. This may also minimise distress for a child who may need to separate from their parents for a specific medical procedure.

Play can help distract a child during a painful medical procedure, for example a puppet could be used to shift the child's focus from the pain of receiving an injection. Language considerations are also important. Young children may be prone to confuse fantasy and reality. When not provided with the appropriate facts, children tend to create a much worse fantasy about a situation than the actual reality. Piaget [21] suggested that children not only confuse fantasy and reality, but the mental and the physical, dreams and reality, and appearance and reality. A child may see someone dressed up as Spiderman and struggle to realise that the person behind the mask is in fact not Spiderman. When young children have been provided with accurate information, they can more accurately imagine it. Trust and respect need to be at the core of our relationships with children. If children are not provided with the truth about what is happening to them, in a developmentally sensitive way, they may feel lied to when they later experience it and then lack trust in professionals in the future.

Therapeutic Play Approaches for Clinical Practice

Play is a universal language. Sadly, adults often forget they can speak the language of play. Play is something we should always tune in to when communicating with and helping children, especially in challenging and anxiety-provoking situations. Play techniques can regularly be incorporated into working with children within the medical arena. Dolls, puppets and figures can help children understand complex situations and help them explain or re-enact how they may be feeling. Medical procedures can be explained using dolls. A child may also use dolls to explain how and where they may be feeling pain or symptoms. By using a doll, puppet or figure provides emotional distance allowing the child to explain something difficult in a way that feels safe by projecting this onto the toy. Puppets can also be used in several ways: children may find it easier to answer difficult questions asked by a puppet than directly from a medical practitioner. A puppet may have its own life story that the child can also ask questions about, which can lead to the child talking about their own story with the puppet.

Having a small play kit in your practice that is inviting is essential. If you are working from an office space, consider a corner dedicated to play that will help a child to feel relaxed. Play will help engage the child and decrease their anxiety, which will lead to a more productive and successful assessment or examination. Helpful things to include in this kit for the school-age child could be Lego bricks, sensory toys such as play doh, bubbles, slime, paper, colouring pens/crayons, puppets, dolls, figures, simple non-competitive games (such as Story Cubes or Story Cards), cuddly toys and soft balls. Sandtrays can also be a great tool when working with children. The sensory nature of sand can help calm children and provide a space for them to play out scenarios and create words. A sandtray could be used to explain and aid the visualisation of a hospital setting. This could help prepare a child for a hospital visit or a medical procedure. You could describe the hospital setting by drawing in the sand and explaining where the children's department is and what they may see when they are there. You could ask the child to pick a figure for themselves so they can walk through the sand in preparation for their upcoming visit. The child may want to choose a strong and courageous animal figure for themselves, like a lion, to help them feel brave towards their upcoming medical event. Alternatively, they may choose a timid creature, like a rabbit, to help externalise and express their fears. Where it may not be possible to use a sandtray, the same activities can be undertaken through drawing tasks or virtual sandtrays. For all children, play is their first language. The more we can use and understand play when communicating with children, the more we will understand them. When it comes to play, children are the professionals, and we must learn and be led by them so we can be the professionals they need.

Parents as Partners

Fostering a good working relationship with parents is vital. Bowlby recognised the importance of supporting parents for positive outcomes for children from the outset noting that 'if a community values its children, it must cherish their parents' [22, pp. 84]. A parent's support for their child is key in supporting healthy development and supporting the child through the challenges that may come with medical care. Respect and authenticity with a nonjudgmental approach are advised when working with parents. Developing a trusting relationship will help activate the trust of the child towards the professional. When children observe positive interactions between their parents and the health professional, it indicates that they are safe.

Considerations for Referral

A child's experiences in their early years will greatly influence their development and functioning in the school years. Identifying concerns as early as possible is key to supporting healthy development. An appointment in a health care setting may be the first opportunity to observe developmental signs that may indicate a need for further referral. A child may attend a medical appointment for a physical ailment where it is also reported that they are struggling with learning, reading, attention, or memory. In this instance the child may need to be referred for a further developmental assessment. Children who have experienced significant medical trauma may also present with feelings of depression, anger or anxiety, where a referral for counselling or therapy may be appropriate.

Chapter Summary

Many important milestones are reached during the school years. Ability, activity and the social world expand significantly. Successful completion of this stage of development results in the virtue of competence. The use of therapeutic play within the health care setting may aid children to develop a sense of industry and self-worth and provide each child with the opportunity to flourish and thrive in the school years, as they navigate the complex world of feelings and relationships.

Reflective Questions and Activities

- Consider how nurturing environments can be created in the health care setting.
- What therapeutic play activities might be appropriate for the school-aged child during a hospital stay?
- How would you incorporate play into an assessment session with a highly anxious child in your practice? How would you 'set the scene'? What therapeutic play techniques might you use?

References

1. Redleaf Quick Guides. (2016). *Developmental milestones of young children*. Redleaf Press.
2. American Heart Association (AHA). (2015). *Overweight in Children*. http://www.heart.org/HEARTORG/GettingHealthy/Overweight-in-Children_UCM_304054_Article.jsp
3. Piaget, J. (2020). *The child's conception of the world*. Alpha Editions.
4. Piaget, J. (1959). *The language and thought of the child* (Vol. 5). Psychology Press.
5. Vygotsky, L. S. (1978). *Mind in society: The development of higher psychological processes*. Harvard University Press.
6. Erikson, E. H. (1997). *The Life Cycle Completed*. WW Norton & Company.
7. Harris, P. L. (1989). *Children and Emotion*. Basil Blackwell.
8. Bowlby, J. (1988). *A Secure Base*. Basic Books.
9. Rubin, K. H., Bukowski, W., & Parker, J. G. (1998). Peer interactions, relationships and groups. In W. Damon & N. Eisenberg (Eds.), *Handbook of child psychology* (pp. 619–700). Wiley.
10. Reavis, R. D. (2007). *Predicting Early Peer Acceptance from Toddler Peer Behavior*. University of North Carolina.
11. Spreen, O., Rissser, A., & Edgell, D. (1995). Developmental neuropsychology. : Oxford University Press. Sternberg, R. J. *Beyond IQ: A triarchic theory of human intelligence*. New York, NY: Cambridge University Press.
12. Markant, J. C., & Thomas, K. M. (2013). Postnatal brain development. In P. D. Zelazo (Ed.), *Oxford handbook of developmental psychology*. Oxford University Press.
13. Siegel, D. J. (2020). *The developing mind third edition: How relationships and the brain interact to shape who we are*. The Guilford Press.
14. Nippold, M. A. (1998). *Later language development: The school-age and adolescent years* (2nd ed.). Pro-Ed.
15. Perry, B. D. (2002). Childhood Experience and the Expression of Genetic Potential: What Childhood Neglect Tells Us About Nature and Nurture. *Brain and Mind, 3*, 79–100.

16. Vygotsky, L. S. (1976). Play and its role in the mental development of the child. In J. Bruner, A. Jolly, & K. Sylva (Eds.), *Play: Its role in development and evolution* (pp. 76–99). Basic Books.
17. Jennings, S. (2018). *Working with Attachment Difficulties in School-Aged Children.* Hinton House.
18. Jennings, S. (2010). *Healthy Attachments and Neuro-Dramatic-Play.* Jessica Kingsley.
19. Stambrook, M., & Parker, K. C. H. (1987). The Development of the Concept of Death in Childhood: A Review of the Literature. *Merrill-Palmer Quarterly, 33*(2), 133–152. http://www.jstor.org/stable/23086325
20. Winnicott, D. (1953). Transitional objects and transitional phenomena. *International Journal of Psychoanalysis, 34,* 89–97.
21. Piaget, J. (1930). *The construction of reality in the child.* Basic Books.
22. Bowlby, J. (1951). *Maternal Care and Mental Health.* World Health Organisation Monograph (serial No.2) Geneva: WHO

Therapeutic Play, Fidelity, and the Adolescent

Phoebe Godfrey, Belinda J. Dean, and Natalie A. Hadiprodjo

Chapter Objectives

At the end of this chapter, you will be able to:

- Outline Erikson's psychosocial framework and the stage of identity versus role confusion for the adolescent.
- Describe holistic play development for the adolescent including the role of play and relationships in shaping the adolescent brain.
- Discuss ethical considerations in working with and supporting the adolescent.
- Highlight how the practitioner can involve parents/caregivers as partners
- Identify principles for playfully engaging adolescents therapeutically in the health care setting.

Introduction

This chapter will provide an overview of the considerations needed as a health care practitioner working with, and caring for, a young person aged between 12 and 18 years. A span of years is defined through the term 'adolescence'. A Future for the World's Children? A WHO-UNICEF-*Lancet* Commission [1] describes adolescence as a critical period of development which results in a window of opportunity for developing agency and identity, but also a time of potential vulnerability. It is a time when negative or positive habits are formed, such as nutrition, exercise and harmful or protective behaviours.

P. Godfrey (✉) · B. J. Dean · N. A. Hadiprodjo
School of Health and Social Development, Deakin University, Geelong, VIC, Australia
e-mail: phoebe.godfrey@deakin.edu.au

Erikson's stages of psychosocial development identify adolescence as a period where the individual faces a conflict of identity versus role confusion [2]. This chapter will explore the possible obstacles an adolescent may face as they work to overcome role confusion and towards an accepted identity and the virtue of fidelity. These years include a range of physical, social, sexual and spiritual changes for the adolescent. Positive resolution of this stage, like those before it, is critical to the development of the personality and the continuing maturity of the adolescent into adulthood [3].

The chapter will explore considerations for nursing and allied health care professionals, with the integration of therapeutic play to support young people and their parents as partners within the health care setting.

Reflection Activity

Consider your own experience of working with adolescents using the following prompts:

- You are to begin working with an adolescent in your health care role. What are your immediate thoughts and feelings?
- Have you worked with adolescents in the past? What was this like?
- How confident are you in working with an adolescent? Are you confident with one age more than another? A particular binary of gender or non-binary status? Certain presentations/difficulties over others?
- What are your 'go-to' strategies to engage and connect with adolescents? Do these differ from those you use when working with younger children?
- What was your own adolescence like? How does your own experience of adolescence inform your view of this stage of life?

Despite adolescence often being perceived as an intimidating developmental stage to engage with, once you understand the adolescent brain, and the developmental conflicts they face, it can ease the self-doubt a professional may have around their capacity to offer support at this age and stage. In this reflection, and the learning to follow, we hope to provide space for you to explore adolescent development and be curious about their world. Simply knowing that they are developing—that they are finding their place in their world and coming into themselves more fully, can be useful to hold in mind, so that you can meet them with kindness and unconditional positive regard.

It can be a scary and overwhelming period for an adolescent, witnessing the physical changes of their body, whilst their brains are rapidly rewiring and reorganising, as they navigate relationships with peers and form their own identities. At the end of the day, adolescents need someone who believes in them, cares for them and accepts them—just as children need at least one person who believes the sun rises and sets with them. Alongside parents, health care professionals can support and form positive connections with adolescents who can help grow their sense of self and establish their identity.

Adolescent Development

Physical and Psychosocial Development

> Of all the stages of life adolescence is the most difficult to describe. Any generalisation about teenagers immediately calls forward an opposite one. Teenagers are maddeningly self-centred, yet capable of impressive acts of altruism. Their attention wanders like a butterfly, yet they can spend hours concentrating on seemingly pointless involvements. They are lazy and rude, yet when you least expect it, they can be loving and helpful [4, p. xiii].

Adolescence is generally associated with the secondary school years, physical maturation and puberty. It is an intense period that when viewed through a psychosocial developmental lens can see an adolescent face a combination of anxiety and pride regarding physical changes (including forming an opinion of body image) and their emerging sexuality [5]. These are just two factors that contribute to an adolescent's developing self-identity. Erikson identified eight stages of psychosocial growth across the lifespan. The stage of development that defines adolescence is the fifth stage, identity versus role confusion. Prior to entering this stage of development, the adolescent needs to successfully navigate the four prior stages (trust versus mistrust, autonomy versus shame and doubt, initiative versus guilt, industry versus inferiority). Each stage of development is characterised by a psychosocial crisis that needs to be overcome and captures potential positive and negative impacts on the personality. Whilst an individual may experience both the positive and the negative elements at each stage, the goal of healthy personality development is to integrate the positive aspects of each stage. The goal for the adolescent is to overcome the challenge of role confusion to establish their identity and independence as they prepare for adulthood.

Erikson [2] recognised that identity formation develops through a recognition of one's abilities, interests, strengths, and weaknesses by both self and others, and is the optimal outcome of a crisis resolution process. A complex process that involves exploration and experimentation to lead to commitment (which Erikson labels as fidelity); through establishing a set of spiritual and religious beliefs; social values including relationships and gender orientation; intellectual and political interests and/or occupation, vocational or career path, as well as culture, ethnicity, and perceptions of one's personality traits—all of which contribute to forming a positive sense of identity [2, 5].

In western cultures, role confusion may be characterised by excessive anxiety and emotional turmoil, seeking independence from parents, or activities previously enjoyed [6], separating self-and/or experimenting with new activities and pleasurable and/or risk-taking behaviours. Exploring new friendships and conforming with a peer group is desired, as the opinion of friends and peers are now highly valued. In collectivist cultures, cultural identity and personal identity need to be considered alongside each other [7]. When considering the importance of social belonging for young people, Goldingay et al. [8] recognise that collectivist traditions such as those of Australian Aboriginal, Torres Strait Islander, and New Zealand Māori cultures identify development as a collectivist process that involves passing cultural knowledge and understanding from the previous generation to the next. They further discuss the importance of identity being formed through oral history sharing including storytelling and time with elders, to learn about connections to land, bloodlines, beliefs, and values for these specific cultures. Western adolescents consider their own story as part of their identity formation which is considered in the literature as developing an autobiographical narrative. Early pretend play development supports this narrative development (see Chap. 4) as adolescents become the holder of their own stories and develop an autobiographical account of past, present, and future [8, 9].

How an adolescent views their physical and sexual development heavily contributes to and impacts on their self-esteem [10]. Powerful influences on an adolescent during this time, include evaluations of others' perceptions of and attitudes towards one's body, and the media (e.g. social media, advertisements, magazines, music videos, video games, movies, and the fashion industry). Difficulties navigating this time of psychosocial development can see one move towards adverse health and social outcomes. These can include psychosocial problems such as eating disorders, depression, and substance misuse or abuse, all of which can contribute to future psychosocial vulnerabilities in adult life.

Carefully targeted access to developmentally appropriately learnings associated with this stage, include an educational focus, exposure to different body types (for example in social media and friendship groups), and an understanding that their feelings and thoughts about their body are not unique to them, but in fact universal at this age, as well as having support from family and friends, and adult mentors who can promote and positively influence the adolescent's adjustment to their bodies. Searching for identity in the period of adolescence is best supported by enabling them to explore parts of themselves, "Who am I?", and the world around them, "Where and how do I fit in?". These two elements, individualistic and contextual components [11], are what enable an adolescent to navigate towards their known and accepted identity.

To support adolescents to achieve a sense of identity, they should be encouraged to explore different roles, opinions, and preferences; be empowered to make choices and reflect on their experiences. They need to be able to explore a variety of activities, relationships, and lifestyles before they can decide and settle on their own viewpoint, set of values, and preferences within life. This process of examining their own perspective, making social comparisons, and evaluating what they know about themselves and what others think of them, supports them in moving towards knowing what makes them unique as an individual. An additional context to consider for adolescent is their online identity. Many adolescents have a digital avatar as well as a modified version of themselves (digital persona) which they choose to share online [12]. Despite positive and negative impacts associated with online versions of self, it is interesting to consider the intersection between adolescents' personal identity and online identity in relation to the adolescent's consideration of self.

Play Development

Play is seen at all ages, stages, abilities, and across cultures. Play does not discriminate; it is a universal language. Many authors describe play in various ways, but there is a united acceptance that play is complex. It can present in all different manners, with a range of resources and toys, or with little to none, it can be a social or an individual task, it can happen in almost any environmental context, primarily allowing the individual to lose a sense of time, and to volunteer their self into their play world. Play develops across the lifespan and may ebb and flow in various formats and intensities. It may look different for a 2-year old compared to a 20-year old. However, play in childhood can be viewed as a precursor to play as a lifetime activity, which contributes to wellness in adulthood and across the lifespan [13].

As shown in the holistic play development diagram (see Chap. 4, Fig. 1), adolescence and Erikson's stage of identity versus role confusion aligns with the later stages of play development as identified by Sue Jennings. The Embodiment-Projection-Role (EPR) paradigm considers the progression of dramatic play in children [14]. This development of EPR is essential for early attachment as well as building a strong base for independence and identity. Integrating EPR through play supports creativity and imagination development and builds opportunities for conflict resolution, resilience, and problem solving, all of which build a strong sense of self [14]. Prendiville [15] explains that any disruptions to this sequential process can impact the child given the influence of the previous stage on the next, however, points out that adults also engage in embodiment, projective, and role play. Adolescents who have missed earlier stages of play development may re-enact these earlier stages to ensure they understand themselves as a separate person (embodiment), understand their emotions, thoughts and become aware of others (projective) and understand relationships and build empathy through seeing the viewpoints of others (role). Within play, the adolescent "can explore and engage in new behaviours and roles, be exposed to different interests, establish likes and dislikes, and socialise with an array of social groups, thereby developing skills, patterns of behaviour, and self-identity" [5, p. 97].

Neurological Development

The holistic play development illustration also shows how adolescence and Erikson's stage of identity versus role confusion align not only with play development but also with brain development. In particular, the development of the more complex parts of the brain such as the cortex, parts of the brain responsible for complex functions such as judgement and decision-making. These higher parts of the brain develop into adulthood and remain plastic throughout life. During adolescence, the brain is also undergoing a period of significant reorganisation, which in part may explain why this stage of life is marked by such intensity. During this stage of development, the brain undergoes structural changes, alongside the growth and pruning of synapses in the brain [16]. The brain develops in a sequential and hierarchical fashion from the lower more primitive parts of the brain responsible for survival, such as the brainstem, to the limbic system or the emotional centre of the brain, through to the thinking brain or cortex [17]. Successful development of these higher regions of the brain relies on the lower parts being provided with positive experiences within the early attachment relationship to shape these foundational parts of the brain. Adverse childhood experiences, such as repeated experiences of trauma, abuse, or neglect, that occur during the development of the lower parts of the brain will impact on the formation of the higher parts of the brain. An adolescent who has experienced adverse childhood experiences may struggle with functions that are managed by the lower brain, such as self-regulation, which in turn will impact on higher brain functions, such as the capacity to empathise and take the perspective of others.

Perry [17] identifies six core strengths of healthy brain development that become possible as the brain develops from the lower parts of the brain up: attachment (making relationships), self-regulation (containing impulses), affiliation (being part of a group), attunement (being aware of others), tolerance (accepting differences), and diversity (valuing differences). For the adolescent, the core strengths of affiliation, attunement, tolerance, and diversity, require experiences that shape a healthy brain across the lifespan. Perry further identifies six R's that comprise positive neurodevelopmental experiences that aid healthy brain development and the strengths above. Experiences must be relevant, repetitive, relational, rhythmic, rewarding, and respectful [18]. Each of these R's can also be applied to the adolescent in the health care setting.

Relevant Therapeutic activities need to be relevant to the area of the brain that you hope to influence. For example, if an adolescent is dysregulated and needs assistance in regulating the lower stress networks of the brain, therapeutic activities need to be relevant to this part of the brain. The lower brain speaks the language of sensation and activities that are somatosensory may be useful to soothe and regulate this part of the brain such as art, music, movement, dance, yoga, or sensory play.

Repetitive The lower brain requires repetition to regulate, this is why music, drumming, dance, and other rhythmic activities have a soothing effect. Furthermore, creating an environment that is predictable with a clear routine, provides structure and a sense of safety. This can be especially important for an adolescent who is facing the uncertainty that comes with medical treatment.

Relational Humans and their brains are born for connection and relationship. Positive relationships with health care professionals will help regulate the stress response system and can help create positive physiological states that support health and healing [19].

Rhythm Refers to the rhythm in a relationship and the importance of attunement. This is especially key in the early attachment relationship or early stages of rapport building. For the adolescent this requires the health care professional to attune and attempt to see the world through their eyes.

Rewarding   This refers to experiences that activate the reward biology in the brain. A key reward hormone is dopamine which can be activated through positive relationships and play. Alternatively, it can also be activated in unhealthy ways through drugs, alcohol, food, self-harm, and risk-taking behaviours [18]. Play is unique as it is closely aligned with the reward pathways in the brain, which is why play is associated with laugher and joy [20].

Respectful   Health care professionals should show respect for an adolescent's racial, cultural, and religious background to further create a sense of safety.

Considerations for Nursing and Allied Health Care

Ethical Considerations

Ethical considerations are paramount for the adolescent client. Considerations around privacy and confidentiality as well as the adolescents' rights (see Chap. 4) need to be at the forefront of the practitioners' thought process when assessing each client. As adolescents work through Erikson's stage of identity versus role confusion, they are developing their sense of self and their place in the world. With this comes fears and anxieties around their self-perception and others' perception of them. They may be afraid to speak about sensitive topics if they do not feel safe and comfortable. Being non-judgemental, showing unconditional positive regard, being fully present and congruent with the adolescent, are core therapeutic skills that build trust and allow the adolescent to feel accepted, and express their concerns fully.

Psychosocial assessments such as the HEEADSSS framework (Home environment, Education and employment, Eating, peer-related Activities, Drugs, Sexuality, Suicide/depression, and Safety) work to maximise communication and minimise judgement. This process occurs by asking open-ended questions that progress from less threatening questions to more intrusive questions to allow the practitioner to build rapport and trust whilst also finding out crucial assessment information [21]. See the following examples from each category:

Home   Who lives with you? What does home mean to you? What would I expect if I came to visit you at home?

Education/Employment   How often are you attending school at the moment? Are you engaged in any employment or making money in any way?

Eating   What do you consider healthy eating to be? Would you say your diet is in line with that? If not, what are the barriers that you can think of?

Activities   What do you do for fun? If you could spend a whole day doing something, what would it be?

Drugs   Does anyone you spend time with drink, smoke, or take any other substances? Do you join in these activities? What would be a typical amount for you to have of this substance?

Sexuality   I wonder if you can tell me about any relationships you have been in or anyone you have dated or had sexual encounters with?

Suicide, Self-harm, and Depression   Do you feel like there is nothing to live for? Do you feel like everything is too hard and you want to give up? Have you ever expressed these feelings to anyone else or really wanted to act on them? Have you found ways of doing things to your body that help to either take the pain away or allow you to feel some pain (stop the numbness?)

Safety   What sort of things help you to feel safe? Is there anyone in your life that helps you to feel safe? Is there anyone in your life who makes you feel unsafe?

When working with an adolescent, just like with any aged client, it is important to establish the boundaries and orientate them to what to expect as a part of this professional relationship. Depending on the age and capacity of the client—this is framed and communicated in different ways—but the end message is the same. You need to establish a safe space that enables you as the health care worker to hold and be with the client—in this case, the adolescent. In addition to maintaining a warm and accepting relationship, one must be clear and communicate the expectations, the importance of confidentiality, privacy, and safety. Where possible it is also important to provide the adolescent with choice.

The following principles can be used when communicating with adolescents:

- Adopt a warm, friendly, and accepting manner.
- Increase feelings of safety by ensuring the adolescent understands privacy and confidentiality.
- Convey feelings of safety using verbal and non-verbal communication such as a gentle voice, and open body language.
- Respect the adolescent's capacity to contribute to their health care needs.
- Offer choice where possible. For example, in relation to their daily schedule (e.g. when to have a shower and when to have visitors), or care requirements (e.g. dressing their own wound with support and taking their own temperature).
- Use empathy and reflect the adolescent's thoughts and feelings in a non-judgemental manner.

For example, an Occupational Therapist introducing themselves to an adolescent patient for the first time may say something like, "Hi John, it's wonderful to meet you. My name is Jenny and I'm an Occupational Therapist. I'm really looking forward to getting to know you. My job is to help you get ready to return home. Some of the things we need to discuss may seem a bit personal. Nothing that you tell me will be shared with anyone else, unless I'm worried that you are at risk of getting hurt, then I will need to share this with other people to keep you safe. I'll be coming to see you every day this week. You have the choice of a morning or afternoon session, what would you prefer?"

Reflective Activity

Using the above principles produce a statement that you could use to introduce yourself to an adolescent client in your current context and role. Consider how you would feel asking this client some of the questions in the HEEADSSS assessment. Practice with a colleague or family member to see how it feels asking these open-ended questions using the guidelines above.

Parents as Partners

As adolescents establish their identity, there may be a tendency to seek independence from their parents/caregivers. It may then be difficult to know how and when to bring parents/caregivers in to further support the adolescent. Just like with younger children, in some cases they may prefer for an adult guardian to be present and close by, and this should always be an option. In instances of medical care, the adolescent may also revisit early stages of development and seek out greater proximity and nurturing from their caregiver. In other cases, an adolescent may be trying to establish their independence and wish to be more autonomous.

Considerations for working with parents/caregivers:

- Know why you need to speak with/engage the parent/caregiver and be transparent about this with the adolescent.
- Invite the adolescent to be present or contribute to parent/caregiver meetings. If they choose to be present, facilitate an open and respectful space where each member has an opportunity to contribute and be heard.

An adult does not have to agree with the adolescent's wants/desires or emotional needs—but should recognise and accept these as important to the adolescent at this present time. Legally, in Australia, mature minors can make their own medical choices so long as they are deemed competent. Generally, the adolescent needs to understand what it is they are consenting to regarding their treatment, what the risks and benefits are, and alternate options [22]. It is ideal to have parents or carers onboard and for transparent communication to occur, however, if it is deemed in the best interest of the adolescent to have treatment (for example commencing contraception) the health care provider and adolescent can determine the best course of action independently without parental consent. This is important to keep in mind when working with adolescents and within a multidisciplinary team. It is also important to consider the adolescent's adult support network, and whether there may be another adult within their network who they feel more comfortable involving for personal support, for example an Aunty/Uncle, or Grandparent. This may be particularly appropriate in collectivist cultures.

The best support an adolescent can receive by the adults in their team, are adults that display consistency, care, and availability [6]. It is often the case that parents/caregivers want to offer advice, and in the process may unintentionally dismiss the adolescent's feelings or perspective and what they view as helpful or problematic. As a health care professional, you can demonstrate a genuine curiosity in the adolescent's perspective and model this for the caregivers.

Therapeutic Play Approaches for Clinical Practice

Although chronologically it is not common for one to think of adolescence as a developmental period of playfulness—play is important to all stages of development. Play provides relive and release and can be a valuable tool for soothing anxiety in the medical setting. With the cognitive shift to formal operational thinking and the increased capacity of adolescents to engage in conversation, be insightful, and use abstract thinking, it is commonly thought that talk-based strategies are most appropriate. However, as was discussed in relation to brain development, adverse childhood experiences, trauma, loss, and grief, may make it difficult for the adolescent to effectively communicate and express their thoughts, feelings, wishes, and needs. Increased emotional conflict at this stage of development may lead the adolescent to be more receptive and better able to communicate and engage in play-based and expressive art activities or therapies [6]. Kottman [23] recognises that there is a limit to cognitive-based therapies for this age range as whilst they may be able to process the content shared, they may have difficulties in finding and choosing words to express the depth of their own experiences, and in viewing multiple perspectives of the more abstract/less tangible experience that the conversation has to offer.

Play and playful approaches support a sense of safety by taking the pressure away from the 'problem,' 'diagnosis', and/or 'fears,' that may exist as a part of the adolescent's medical or treatment journey. Play can also increase positive emotions and lift the adolescent's spirits. Play and expressive art activities can support an individual who may need to communicate without words, but can describe their own creations, and can hence offer insight into the metaphor of their experience. Conversation may or may not be present during these activities. Sometimes free expression, being in nature, or having some music on during these tasks can be beneficial [24]. Consideration should also be given to mobility restrictions due to a medical condition, surgery, or other difficulties when planning therapeutic play activities.

Within a medical setting technology may be especially suitable given its accessibility. Technology offers adolescence a world of resources for emotional and self-expression, social engagement, communication, and connection. Fear often exists surrounding the digital and virtual reality worlds of the 'unknown' [25], but when used in intentional and positive ways, they can support adolescents, particularly in a health care setting where access to more traditional expressive resources may be limited due to space, noise disturbance, and/or hygiene concerns. The digital and virtual reality worlds can offer experiences such as photography, photo stories or blogging, videography, free expression through mandalas, virtual colouring and painting, guided imagery, or meditation apps such as those offered through Smiling Mind and Headspace or the VR apps such as Tripp, Virtual Sandtray app, or other printed materials such as blank comic stories pages see picklebums, or interactive games such as Rory's story cubes (including the medic version) [26].

Consideration for Referral

As has been identified across this chapter, adolescence constitutes a time in which the individual faces significant neurological, physical, social, and emotional changes and experiences as they work towards forming their own identity. Some adolescents will face specific issues such as depression and suicidal thoughts and/or idealisation, self-harm, body image issues, and/or drug/alcohol abuse. These issues warrant referral to specialist support so that the individual may be best supported to overcome these challenges and move towards finding and accepting their own identity.

Chapter Summary

This chapter has provided an overview of adolescence as viewed through Erikson's psychosocial stage of identity versus role confusion, highlighting the conflicts and challenges an adolescent may face on their path to identity formation. Genuine care, openness, and respect for the adolescent will increase the adolescent's feelings of safety, trust, and comfort across their health care journey. Knowing when, and how to engage other significant adults, including parents and caregivers as partners, as well as utilising developmentally appropriate playful approaches will support positive health outcomes for the adolescent.

Reflective Questions and Activities

- Take a large piece of paper and create a body outline on a large sheet of butcher's paper. Take some time to brainstorm experiences in adolescence that may lead to identity formation. Write these inside the body outline. Next brainstorm experiences in adolescence that may lead to role confusion and list these experiences outside of the body outline.

- Now that you have completed this chapter and the reflective exercises throughout, how would you now rate your confidence in working with adolescents?
- What is one strategy that you can apply to your current context or health care practice?

References

1. Clark, H., Coll-Seck, A. M., Banerjee, A., Peterson, S., Dalglish, S. L., Ameratunga, S., et al. (2020). A future for the world's children? A WHO–UNICEF–Lancet Commission. *Lancet, 395*(10224), 605–658. https://www.thelancet.com/journals/lancet/article/PIIS0140-6736(19)32540-1/fulltext
2. Erikson, E. H. (1980). *Identity and the life cycle*. W.W Norton and Company.
3. Lerwick, J. L. (2013). Psychosocial implications of pediatric surgical hospitalization. *Seminars in Pediatric Surgery, 22*(3), 129–133. https://doi.org/10.1053/j.sempedsurg.2013.04.003
4. Csikszentmihalyi, M., & Larson, R. (1984). *Being adolescent: conflict and growth in the teenage years*. Basic Books.
5. Vroman, K. (2010). In transition to adulthood: the occupations and performance skills of adolescents. In J. Case-Smith & J. C. O'Brien (Eds.), *Occupational therapy for children* (Vol. 6, pp. 84–107). Elsevier Health Sciences.
6. Smith, J. E., & Michero, E. (2016). The extraordinary 12-year-old. In D. C. Ray (Ed.), *A Therapist's guide to child development: the extraordinarily Normal years*. Routledge.
7. Schwartz, S. J., Zamboanga, B. L., & Weisskirch, R. S. (2008). Broadening the study of the self: integrating the study of personal identity and cultural identity. *Social and Personality Psychology Compass, 2*(2), 635–651. https://doi.org/10.1111/j.1751-9004.2008.00077.x
8. Goldingay, S., Stagnitti, K., Dean, B., Robertson, N., Francis, E., & Davidson, D. (2020). *Storying beyond social difficulties with neuro-diverse adolescents: the 'Imagine, create, Belong' Social Development Program*. Routledge.
9. Stagnitti, K. (2021). *Learn to play therapy: principles, process and practical activities* (2nd ed.). Learn to Play.
10. Sanstrock, J. W. (2003). *Adolescence (9)*. McGraw-Hill Higher Education.
11. Kunnen, E. S., Bosma, H. A., & VanGeert, P. L. C. (2001). A dynamic systems approach to identity formation: theoretical background and methodological possibilities. In J. E. Nurmi (Ed.), *Navigating through adolescences: European perspectives* (pp. 251–278). Routledge Falmer.
12. Faccennini, F. (2021). Digital avatars: thinking about personal identity in social media. *Philosophy Today, 65*(3), 599–617. https://doi.org/10.5840/philtoday2021520409
13. Brown, S., & Vaughan, C. (2009). *Play. How it shapes the brain, opens the imagination, and invigorates the soul*. Scribe Publications.
14. Jennings, S. (2014). Applying an embodiment-projection-role framework in groupwork with children. In J. Howard & E. Prendiville (Eds.), *Play therapy today: contemporary practice with individuals, groups, and carers* (pp. 81–96). Routledge.
15. Prendiville, E. (2021). The EPR informed psychotherapist. In E. Prendiville & J. Parson (Eds.), *Clinical applications of the therapeutic powers of play: case studies in child and adolescent psychotherapy*. Routledge.
16. Badenoch, B. (2008). *Being a brain-wise therapist: a practical guide to interpersonal neurobiology (Norton series on interpersonal neurobiology)*. WW Norton & Company.

17. Perry, B. (2009). Examining child maltreatment through a neurodevelopmental lens: clinical applications of the neurosequential model of therapeutics. *Journal of Loss & Trauma, 14*(4), 240–255. https://doi.org/10.1080/15325020903004350

18. Gaskill, R. L. (2019). Neuroscience helps play therapists go low so children can aim high. *International Journal of Play Therapy, 25*(1), 8–10.

19. Ludy-Dobson, & Perry, B. D. (2010). The role of healthy relational interactions in buffering the impact of childhood trauma. In E. Gil (Ed.), *Working with children to heal interpersonal trauma: the power of play* (pp. 26–43). Guilford Press.

20. Panksepp, J., & Biven, L. (2012). *The archaeology of mind: neuroevolutionary origins of human emotions*. W. W. Norton & Co.

21. Goldenring, J. M., & Rosen, D. S. (2004). Getting into adolescent heads: An essential update. *Contemporary Pediatrics-Montvale, 21*(1), 64–92.

22. Levy, N. B. L. (2018). *Legal issues...Maintaining confidentiality: Minors*. CINAHL Nursing Guide.

23. Kottman, T. (2011). *Play therapy basics and beyond*. American Counseling Association.

24. Flahive, M. W., & Ray, D. (2007). The effect of group sandtray therapy with preadolescents. *Journal for Specialists in Group Work, 32*(4), 362–382.

25. Goodwin, K. (2016). *Raising your child in a digital world*. Finch Books.

26. Parson, J., & Renshaw, K. (2018). *Engaging adolescents using therapeutic play and creative arts*. Deakin University short course.

Part III

Case Presentations

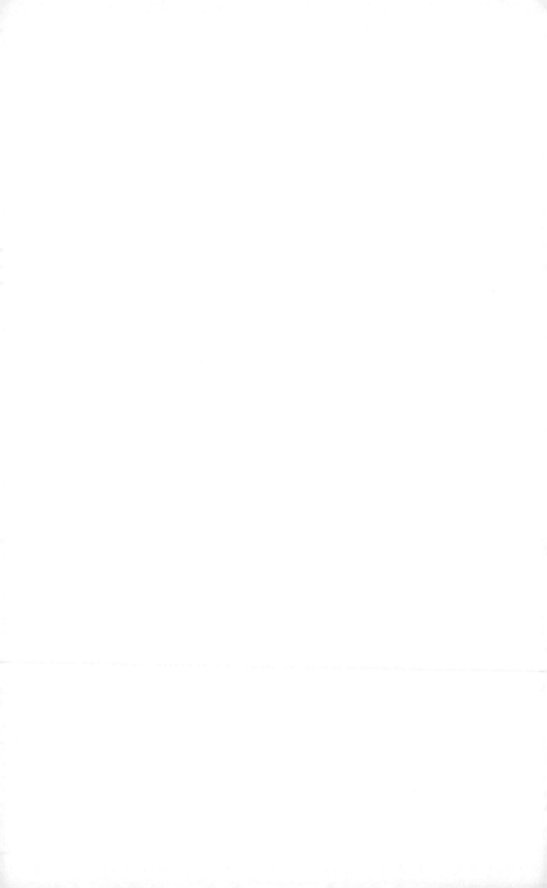

Preparing Jess for an Allergy Assessment

Michelle Perrin

Objectives

At the end of this chapter, you will be able to:

- Understand the importance of the therapeutic relationship in the process of re-framing traumatic experiences.
- Consider the unique needs of the child and family in developing individual coping plans.
- Develop awareness of strategies to support children and young people during needle-related procedures.

Introduction

If you are distressed by anything external, the pain is not due to the thing itself; but to your estimate of it; and this you have the power to revoke at any moment—Marcus Aurelius

There is an increasing prevalence of asthma and allergic disease in children and young people [1]. It is estimated that around 20% of the global population are impacted by asthma, allergic rhinitis, atopic dermatitis, or food allergies [2]. Symptoms and severity of disease vary; however, it is understood that for many there is a significant psychosocial impact and reduced quality of life [2, 3].

M. Perrin (✉)
John Hunter Children's Hospital, Newcastle, NSW, Australia
e-mail: michelle.perrin@health.nsw.gov.au

© The Author(s), under exclusive license to Springer Nature
Switzerland AG 2022
J. A. Parson et al. (eds.), *Integrating Therapeutic Play Into Nursing and Allied Health Practice*, https://doi.org/10.1007/978-3-031-16938-0_11

The immune system is composed of organs, cells, and proteins throughout the body. It is responsible for fighting infections and protecting the body. Immunology and Allergy Specialists diagnose and treat a range of Immunology disorders including those stemming from underactive immune systems (immunodeficiencies); and overactive immune responses, such as allergies and auto-immune disorders. Children at risk of serious illness or with severe symptoms may require hospital visits; regular outpatient appointments; and frequent treatments to assist in managing symptoms [4]. Treatment varies, however, there are some common interventions, such as skin prick testing (for allergies); immunotherapy, to manage symptoms relating to allergic disease; venipuncture; oral food challenges; oral and intra-dermal drug challenges; and dressing routines to manage eczema. In this chapter, we look at Jess' experience with allergen immunotherapy (AIT) and venipuncture. AIT results in a reduction of symptoms to allergy as tolerance is developed through regular, increasing doses of allergen extract. AIT can be delivered by regular injection or, in some cases daily oral medication [5]. In Jess' case, she attends the Allergy and Immunology outpatient clinic monthly for injection to manage severe allergic rhinitis.

The Allergy and Immunology team provides both inpatient and outpatient services. We are composed of two Consultant Immunologist's, a rotating Registrar, a Clinical Nurse Consultant (CNC), two Clinical Nurse Specialists (CNS), Dietitian, Child Life Therapist (CLT), and administrative staff. My role as the Child Life Therapist involves supporting children and families through their healthcare experience; to develop strategies to engage in and manage treatment and support ongoing child development.

We notice that several children present to clinic with anxiety—due to previous healthcare experiences; relating to their disease; and in some cases, generalised to their daily life. Many parents of children with severe food allergies describe feelings of anxiety, especially around accidental exposure. This is not surprising given the degree of vigilance that is required to prevent such exposures. Patel et al. described children with food allergies, and their families as being significantly impacted emotionally, socially, and financially [6]. Others support this view and purport that separation anxiety in children with food allergies is experienced to a greater degree than siblings without food allergy [7]. A recent study has shown that there is an increased psychosocial impact for children who have had two or more exposures in the past year; and those whose parents have reported anxiety [8]. It is recommended that clinicians screen for anxiety and provide appropriate support and referrals [6, 9]. The Child Life Therapist supports children with anxiety or distress in the context of their medical condition and treatments. Children and families whose lives are significantly impacted are provided with referrals to external services such as psychology, play therapy, or counsellors.

Introducing Jess

Jess was referred to Child Life Therapy by an Immunologist for commencement of monthly immunotherapy injections. These injections will continue for around 3 years and occasional blood tests will be required. When I met Jess, she was almost 7 years old, she lives with her parents and two siblings in a small rural community around 1 ½ h from the hospital. She spent a short time in the neonatal intensive care unit (NICU) at birth and has had two hospital admissions via emergency departments for regular childhood accidents and illness. The Immunologist was concerned that injections would not be tolerated as Jess had been apprehensive at her last skin prick test and had described her fear of needles as 'off the scale'. The Immunologist described Jess as a delightful young girl who was able to clearly articulate her worries. Jess has been diagnosed with a sensory processing disorder. There has been discussion about assessment for autism spectrum disorder with their GP, however, the family felt that Jess was managing and did not feel it to be necessary at this point.

The Clinical Setting

This case study evolves in a tertiary hospital with a large catchment area providing specialist paediatric services to children and young people from regional and rural areas. It is attached to an adult's hospital, sharing some of the services such as radiology, emergency, pathology, and operating theatres. There is a great deal of activity with staff, patients, and visitors moving hurriedly about, the buzz of coffee machines in the cafeterias contributing to the cacophony of sounds, bright lights, big open spaces with high ceilings, and a myriad of smells. It is no wonder that some visitors describe a sense of feeling overwhelmed.

Visitors enter the hospital beside the emergency department and make their way past pathology to attend children's outpatient clinics. Before arriving for their appointment, they will have walked past two areas that have the potential to trigger an unpleasant memory. Families sit in the waiting room, sometimes for an extended period. This space was designed with consideration to a paediatric population; however, it is a large open space, with bays of fixed seating, and limited access to appropriate toys. This area does not contribute to soothing or calming an aroused child. Clinic rooms are neutral in colour, have a treatment bed, desk with computer where the clinician sits, and chairs for the patient and family. The environment, uniforms, and general order to this scenario serves important functionality, however, each of these subtle messages communicate an imbalance of power, and resultant loss of control for patients and families [10]. As space is limited, Child Life Therapist's often see children in these clinic rooms, sometimes with others coming and going. Goodyear-Brown poses the question of whether the therapeutic space communicates felt safety that is required for children to take risks, leading to growth [11]. As described above, there are obvious challenges to providing this felt safety in the healthcare environment and to do this each child's unique needs must be considered.

Activity one: Refer to end of the chapter for further exploration of the impact of the healthcare environment.

Assessment

Gathering as much information as possible to inform interventions is essential to build a care plan that supports each child and family. A care plan should have the goal of building resilience and minimising the potential for iatrogenic trauma [12].

Each child and family bring with them important stories that provide insight into the development of their own coping plan. A child's temperament, level of anxiety, exposure to medical procedures, parental stress, and parental support, all influence how a child responds to their illness and treatment [13]. Assessment can take many forms and should consider all perspectives. The 'Emotional Safety Framework' [12] explores a comprehensive approach to risk assessment for medical stress and lists a range of formalised assessments, such as the Psychosocial Risk Assessment in Pediatrics (PRAP) tool [13].

Reflection
Often, Child Life Therapists find themselves pressured to 'come and fix things', when the child is already in the procedure room distressed. As my practice has evolved, I have gained the confidence to insist on a pause in treatment to allow a thorough assessment and to plan appropriate interventions. Of course, there are times due to urgent clinical concerns, it is not possible to wait. In these moments it is essential to make decisions quickly with the patient and family, communicate the plan to the team, and to advocate for adequate sedation if required. Debriefing with the child, and family as well as staff should not be overlooked in these situations and follow-up interventions to process the medical procedure should be supported.

Activity two: Refer to end of chapter to consider assessment and interventions for a toddler requiring a blood test.

Learning More about Jess

Prior to meeting Jess, I gathered information from a variety of sources to help me plan for our first meeting in clinic. These included:
1. Discussion with familiar clinicians to provide insight into coping and engagement.
   Clinicians explained that Jess had taken a long time to come around to agreeing to skin prick testing—she had a lot of questions and sought

control by wanting to feel the lancet herself. Jess did agree to the procedure and watched whilst it occurred.

2. Reviewed previous medical notes and correspondence.

   There was limited information in previous notes that described her coping with hospitalisation despite her mother reporting difficult experiences in the emergency department 2 years prior.

   Jess was on a waiting list for a urology appointment due to frequent night-time enuresis.

3. Phone conversation with Jess' mother.

   Jess' mother was keen to engage and reported that Jess has a diagnosed sensory processing disorder. She attends mainstream schooling, achieving well academically. She has some difficulty engaging socially with peers but has a small group of like-minded friends. She has been described as hyperactive and has occasional aggressive outbursts at school and home which appear to be in response to being overwhelmed or bored.

   She has had seven blood tests in the past 2 years, all of which she has been restrained for in local pathology services. She has a background of asthma, and eczema, which is well managed. Her mother was concerned about the immunotherapy injections and felt that she would be best told on the morning of the visit given her likelihood to become more distressed.

   Due to visitor restrictions relating to COVID-19 only one family member could attend clinic. It was decided that Jess would attend with her father. There were no specific calming tools that the family identified when Jess became overwhelmed. It was suggested that she would need time to ask questions and would enjoy exploring sensory and fidget toys. In this conversation, I reiterated the process of immunotherapy injections. It is important that the carer has a good understanding of what will occur, so they provide accurate information to the child.

Reflection

When talking with Jess' mother I became curious as to whether her repeated exposure to distressing medical procedures was contributing to her bedwetting and her tendencies for impulsive aggression, hyperactivity, and social withdrawal. My learning around trauma suggested that her internal alarm system might be in overdrive, making it difficult to remain in emotional control [14, 15].

Building the Foundation—The Therapeutic Relationship

'There is no greater agony than bearing an untold story inside you'—Maya Angelou

There is much discussion in the literature around the emotional effects of medical procedures on children if not well managed:

- Early medical experiences leave an imprint on children, and a trauma response may be elicited when a child feels helpless, perhaps magnified if they were restrained [14].
- Frightening experiences in healthcare, such as undergoing painful or distressing procedures can cause treatment-related, or iatrogenic trauma [16].
- Medical procedures can be stored as traumatic emotional memories [17].

It could be assumed that given Jess' admission to NICU, and repeated frightening medical experiences involving restraint, that there was potential for medical traumatic stress.

The therapeutic relationship is perhaps the most vital aspect in supporting a child who has experienced medical traumatic stress. McInnes describes how Anna Freud, believed that children were able to play out their unconscious thoughts and discuss their conscious thoughts in the context of a facilitated environment and therapeutic relationship [18]. The therapeutic relationship develops in the presence of the three core conditions of empathy, congruence, and unconditional positive regard. These conditions were first introduced by Carl Rogers as some of the necessary conditions for change to occur [19, 20].

This relationship is important in the context of the medical environment as children can easily become hyper-aroused, or hypo-aroused when triggered by sounds, sights, and smells of equipment that has previously caused distress. When they become dysregulated and do not feel safe, they lose the capacity to engage [21]. In the face of potential danger, the vagal nerve prepares us to fight or flee. In this stress response, we are not able to utilise our brain's full potential and require co-regulation [22]. The sensitive therapist can co-regulate the child and support them to expand their window of tolerance—the space in which they remain regulated and can function effectively [23], increasing their capacity to cope.

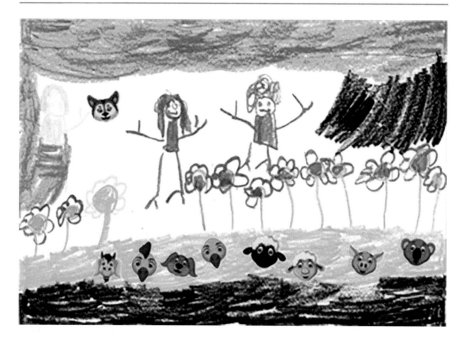

Drawing by 'Jess'—"Us playing together whilst Dad waits'

Meeting Jess

I had many questions around what happened to Jess, and how that would shape our time together. I was armed with a range of fidget and other sensory items to explore and was looking forward to building a relationship that I was hoping would, over time, support a change in her perception of treatment. I found a young girl sitting next to her father, picking at her fingernails, eyes downcast, repeatedly scanning the room, taking in all who entered. I sensed a frightened child who was on high alert for danger. To support her need for safety I positioned myself on the floor, allowing plenty of space between us. Jess made eye contact with me when I introduced myself.

She quickly noticed the sensory toys and reached out for one. At that moment, a nurse entered the room and Jess' eyes darted to the door, noticing the yellow kidney dish she was holding. Jess moved under the chair, clutching the legs and began to scream 'she's got the needle, she's going to hurt me'. The nurse withdrew from the room, however, Jess remained in this position repeating her mantra. In this moment I noticed that her father remained calm and gently reached down placing his hand on her back. This act showed me that he was a supportive presence, and he was demonstrating that he was with her in this moment.

Jess remained highly aroused for some time, we moved rooms to give us space and lessen her perceived threat. Jess held on to the chair as we moved, keeping a physical barrier from danger. The team were in agreeance that we needed to provide a safe and positive first experience of immunotherapy to influence future interventions and reduce the chance of further trauma. They were fortunately supportive of time, allowing myself and her father to assist in regulating her back to a safe place.

I continued to play with the sensory toys, commenting on the textures as I went. Jess slowly released a hand from the chair and picked up a slime ball set inside a net, squeezing it hard and pounding it into the floor. Tracking her motions as we went, she returned her gaze to me, and I validated her fear. 'You felt frightened when the nurse brought the needle into the room'. Jess quietly nodded.

Interventions

Play relating to a child's medical experience allows them the opportunity to share their story, gain empowerment, experiment with different endings and re-interpret traumatic experiences [24]. Early developmental theorists Freud, and Erikson both valued the use of play in processing traumatic events to gain meaning and control [18]. Loose parts play, which can include a range of medical equipment as well as any other resources available, such as craft supplies or items found in nature, allows children the opportunity to gain mastery and empowerment in a creative and fun way. Children can learn about their illness or treatment and experiment, creating meaning out of their healthcare experience [25]. Using the skills of tracking and empathic responding the therapist can facilitate a child-centred approach to medical play allowing the child to feel acceptance and unconditional positive regard, enabling an environment in which to express whatever they would like to explore in their play [26].

When facilitating medical or traumatic play it is important to be mindful that even play experiences and discussions may trigger a significant emotional response and should be titrated to support the child's coping.

Charles Schaefer defines the 'Therapeutic Powers of Play' in four domains—Facilitates Communication, Fosters Emotional Wellness, Enhances Social Relationships, and Increases Personal Strengths [27]. Many of these core agents of change were enacted with Jess. I draw attention to the category of 'Fostering Emotional Wellness' where he describes the agents of change as catharsis, counter-conditioning of fears, abreaction, positive emotions, stress inoculation, and stress management. Our play experiences enabled Jess to gain control in the environment and take charge of her fear which is essential to make change [28].

Due to distance from the hospital and COVID-19 restrictions, I was only able to see Jess on the days of her injection. I gathered some resources for her and her parents to explore creatively together at home with some instructions for the parents on supporting child-led play. Jess decided I needed homework as well and asked that we both create something to show each other on her next visit. We were both allowed to collect any loose parts we pleased. This served the purpose of Jess gaining some control with equipment she may have previously avoided and strengthened our therapeutic relationship, fostering positive emotions in her wanting to return to the hospital to see my creation.

Jess required a blood test shortly after she commenced immunotherapy. Prior to this we spent 1 h together to build our 'plan of attack' (Jess' words). There was a selection of sensory, creative, construction, imaginary, and medical play items available to Jess. She began by building a fort out of large blocks to play inside of. We had to retrieve extra blocks to make the walls high enough for her to hide (containment). Jess and I sat inside, and she initiated medical play using a calico doll. Jess re-enacted blood tests on the doll, frequently getting them 'wrong', which made the doll angry. Jess would facilitate the doll crashing the walls of the fort when this happened. Tracking and empathic responding was used to support Jess in this play and to assist her to gain some meaning—"He (the doll) is mad they didn't get it right again! I wonder what would help them to make it right?'. There were points of play interruption in which Jess got up to dance and would return to the play. We were able to develop our plan of things we could do, and what we could ask the blood collectors to do to 'get it right'.

Reflection
Jess had the option to pause the play when she needed. The play interruptions of dancing involved jumping, twirling, and highly physical movements. I felt that this was her instinctive way of using rhythmic movements for brainstem regulation when she became overwhelmed.

Strategies to Support Needle-Related Procedures

There are many and varied strategies to support children and young people requiring needle-related procedures. The key message would be to ensure a comprehensive assessment is undertaken to inform what may be useful for each child.

Like adults, children (even some young infants) and young people have different coping styles. Some prefer to attend to what is happening to feel in control and prefer a calm and supportive person to break down the steps and talk them through, drawing attention to the procedure. Others respond better to diversion or refocusing strategies.

It is beneficial to develop a procedure plan with children in advance. This should be discussed when the child is in a calm, regulated state. The child, family, or healthcare worker should communicate this plan to the team involved for a coordinated approach. Those developing the plan with the child must be aware of the choices that can be followed through in the specific clinical environment.

Strategies that can be employed to support children include, but are not limited to:

- Sensory considerations such as the use of topical anaesthetic creams; cooling or vibration devices to alter the sensation of the needle.
- Regulated breathing techniques that stimulate the parasympathetic nervous system.
- Distraction techniques carefully planned with the child and carer.
- Virtual reality as a diversion or designed to support coping through the procedure.
- Guided imagery.
- Hypnotic pain management technique—such as the magic glove [29], guided by a trained clinician.
- Deciding on a position of comfort in which the child can maintain contact with their primary carer whilst maintaining a safe environment.
- Planning who will be the primary voice that the child can focus on.
- Breaking the procedure down into small, achievable steps, to make it more manageable if a child is overwhelmed.
- Encouraging participation when appropriate and desired (e.g. removing own numbing cream or placing the tourniquet).

All discussions with the child should be honest and consider what the child may experience from a sensory perspective.

On our first meeting, Jess told me 'I feel things bigger than other people'. She described being bothered by loud or sudden noises, sometimes clothes felt funny on her body, she didn't like feeling hot, and sometimes she would cry at things that others might not—like having a needle. She described her heart starting to beat fast and feeling sweaty when she thought about needles. After engaging in some grounding activities Jess removed the chair she had kept as a barrier and said she was ready to talk about the needle. She told me that she wanted to do it because she wanted her symptoms to go away.

We explored a range of sensory options to alter the sensation of the injection, such as the Buzzy® [30] and the use of topical anaesthetic. Jess enjoyed the vibrating sense of the Buzzy®, however, preferred to hold it in her opposite hand as a distraction during the injection. She preferred not to use the topical anaesthetic cream as she did not like the feeling of this being applied.

We used a range of sensory activities to support the regulation of emotions prior to injections. Sometimes we would jump down the corridor to give Jess the proprioceptive feedback she required. Over time Jess was able to initiate her own breathing techniques to support her injections. On the first two occasions she required much support to remain in her window of tolerance. She sat on her father's lap and cried, although remained in control. On the fourth injection she asked her father to sit beside her. Jess was in control of the timing of this step-down of support and felt empowered to make these decisions. By the sixth injection she was sitting alone, and we celebrated this achievement of the goal that she had set for herself.

Each month, we would close our time by her writing a letter to herself for her next injection. She focused on what had helped as a reminder that she was safe. This was a powerful tool as it used her own words to describe her feelings and progress.

Reflection

I was impressed by Jess' interoceptive awareness. She clearly articulated the feelings within her body as her stress response was activated. Due to her internal attunement, we could quickly identify and engage strategies for regulation. Jess has taught me to focus on this awareness when working with other children in dysregulated states and to engage in my own strategies when feeling overwhelmed.

Activity three: See end of the chapter. What self-care strategies support you to work with children and families in stressful situations?

Jess' father joked that she saved up every story from her month to share with me when she arrived. She often brought items of importance to show me. I protected the time for this sharing. This was key to maintaining our therapeutic relationship and demonstrated the core conditions of empathy, congruence, and unconditional positive regard. It was important to demonstrate to Jess that I was an ally, even if she had a difficult time with her injection.

Where to Next?

Our objective is always to empower the family with strategies for managing procedures and the capacity to advocate for their own care. It is pleasing to report that Jess now attends her monthly injections independently. She has been able to cope with adjustments to treatment such as an unfamiliar nurse administering the injection. I make a point of dropping in occasionally, to maintain the therapeutic relationship. She feels confident in her injections but has requested support for her blood tests when required.

The family are considering a recommendation to pursue Play Therapy or Psychology in the community. We are fortunate to have a small amount of funding for Child Life Therapy services for this cohort of patients, however, the scope must remain within the context of medical treatment. It became apparent throughout our time together that Jess would benefit from these services to help her in understanding and managing her big emotions and sensory experiences.

Learning Activities and Reflective Questions

Activity One

Consider a busy emergency department. There are many adults and children in a large, noisy, brightly lit waiting area. There is uncertainty about wait times. Inside the paediatric area you are allocated a bedspace with curtains as the boundaries. Around you are other children and young people being treated for a variety of illness and injuries. Everyone is wearing masks due to the increased risk of COVID-19 infection, it is difficult to identify staff and their roles due to protective clothing.

List some of the things you may see, hear, smell, touch, and taste.

Now imagine this as a 7-year-old child who has difficulties processing sensory experiences.

How May the Child Present?

Hyper- and hypo-arousal can present in a variety of ways. Some may include:

- Person appearing withdrawn, quiet, or seemingly unresponsive, motionless.
- Overly vigilant of the environment—awareness of background noises, staff and visitor movements, equipment in the environment.
- Acute responses to noise, light, touch, and other stimuli.
- Aggression.
- Inability to be still—seeking regulation through physical activity.

What Would Enable them to Feel a Sense of Safety in this Environment?

- Capacity to remain close to primary caregiver.
- Introduction to staff members and their role.
- Developmentally appropriate information about the treatment plan.
- Capacity to make meaningful choices.

- Ability to control some elements of the environment such as cubicle lighting during waiting periods, and blankets for warmth.
- Access to comforting items and opportunity to engage in familiar activities whilst waiting.

Activity Two

Consider how you could quickly assess and prepare a toddler for a blood test.

What Information Would Be Important to Inform your Interventions?

- Is there a primary caregiver available to support? How are they feeling about the procedure? Do they require support or education?
- Has the child experienced similar medical interventions in the past? How did they respond? Was there anything that helped?
- How would the parent or carer normally provide comfort if the toddler was upset or unsettled?
- Does the child suck their thumb for comfort? If so which one? Use this to advocate for appropriate location of blood test.
- Have the staff considered topical anaesthetics such as numbing cream and cooling devices?
- What words have the carers used to inform the child of their illness or injury?

How Could You Assess and Prepare the Carer for Their Role in the Procedure?

- Establish carers coping. Have they had challenging experiences with similar procedures? Do they require support to remain regulated? NB: If the carer needs to debrief their own experience this should be done away from the child.
- Provide information on what they can do to help, such as be an active participant in diversion activities, regulating calm breathing, stroking, singing, and soothing.
- Rehearse a position of comfort that allows the carer to support their child and maintain physical contact.
- Rehearse phrases to support coping and validate the child's concerns.

What Might the Toddler and Carer Experience from a Sensory Perspective?

- Bright lights of procedure room.
- Temperature change—some people report feeling cold in procedure room.
- Tightness of tourniquet.

- Cold, wet sensation of cleaning wipe.
- Smell of cleaning and remove wipes that assist with tape removal.
- Firm touch and holding of arm whilst looking for the vein and throughout the procedure.
- Multiple voices and instructions.
- Seeing equipment for procedure and other items in the room, some of which may be unfamiliar.
- Sharpness of injection, feeling of pressure as needle is inserted, feeling of needle being removed.
- Seeing blood in the tubes, and possibly on the bed.
- Hearing the familiar voice of the carer.

Consider Some Ways You May Be Able to Support and Prepare them for this

- Rehearse the procedure on a doll if time permits. Allow the child to explore the tourniquet, wipes, tapes, cotton balls, and blood tubes.
- Explain why this needs to happen in a developmentally appropriate way. Extend on information already provided by carers, such as 'Mummy tells me your tummy has been feeling sore, this will help us to work out why'.
- Spend some time building a trusting relationship, this can be done quickly by establishing toddler's interests or favourite activities.
- Establish any comfort items such as a favourite blanket, dummy, or soft toy that could be used for a pleasurable and familiar sensation.
- Encourage carer to participate in ways that they are comfortable, such as singing a familiar song, stroking, or reading a story.
- Discuss the importance of one voice in the procedure room and decide with the clinicians who this will be.
- Introduce and trial non-pharmacological supports such as cooling and vibration that may provide alternative sensory input and assist with pain [30, 31].
- Remove any unnecessary equipment from the procedure room.
- Have the room prepared prior to child entering the treatment space.

Activity Three

Child Life Therapists who support children during medical procedures support children to safely express and contain big emotions. At times, the therapist may experience compassion fatigue and require time to process their own big emotions. It is essential that self-care is seen as a priority.

List some of the signs you notice in your own body at times of stress.

What activities do you engage in to regulate your stress response?

Some Helpful Resources

https://www.healthcaretoolbox.org/
   https://emotional-safety.org/emotional-safety-in-pediatrics/
   https://paincarelabs.com/buzzy/
   https://www.verywellmind.com/abdominal-breathing-2584115
   https://pediatric-pain.ca/wp-content/uploads/2013/04/The_Magic_Glove12.pdf

References

1. Osborne, N. J., Koplin, J. J., Martin, P. E., Gurrin, L. C., Thiele, L., Tang, M. L., et al. (2010). The HealthNuts population-based study of paediatric food allergy: Validity, safety and acceptability. *Clinical and Experimental Allergy: Journal of the British Society for Allergy and Clinical Immunology, 40*(10), 1516–1522. https://doi.org/10.1111/j.1365-2222.2010.03562.x

2. Dierick, B. J. H., van der Molen, T., Flokstra-de Blok, B. M. J., Muraro, A., Postma, M. J., Kocks, J. W. H., & van Boven, J. F. M. (2020). Burden and socioeconomics of asthma, allergic rhinitis, atopic dermatitis and food allergy. *Expert review of pharmacoeconomics & outcomes research, 20*(5), 437–453. https://doi.org/10.1080/14737167.2020.1819793

3. Nowak-Wegrzyn, A., Hass, S. L., Donelson, S. M., Robison, D., Cameron, A., Etschmaier, M., et al. (2021). The Peanut allergy burden study: Impact on the quality of life of patients and caregivers. *World Allergy Organization Journal, 14*(2). https://doi.org/10.1016/j.waojou.2021.100512

4. Australian Society of Clinical Immunology and Allergy (ASCIA). (2019). Hay fever (allergic rhinitis): fast facts Retrieved from https://allergy.org.au/images/pcc/ff/ASCIA_Hay_Fever_Fast_Facts_2019.pdf

5. Australian Society of Clinical Immunology and Allergy (ASCIA). (2020). Allergen Immunotherapy (AIT) FAQ (Frequently Asked Questions).

6. Patel, N., Herbert, L., & Green, T. D. (2017). The emotional, social, and financial burden of food allergies on children and their families. *Allergy and asthma proceedings, 38*(2), 88–91. https://doi.org/10.2500/aap.2017.38.4028

7. King, R. M., Knibb, R. C., & Hourihane, J. O. B. (2009). Impact of peanut allergy on quality of life, stress and anxiety in the family. *Allergy, 64*(3), 461–468. https://doi.org/10.1111/j.1398-9995.2008.01843.x

8. Acaster, S., Gallop, K., Vries, J., Ryan, R., Vereda, A., & Knibb, R. C. (2020). Peanut allergy impact on productivity and quality of life (PAPRIQUA): Caregiver-reported psychosocial impact of peanut allergy on children. *Clinical & Experimental Allergy, 50*(11), 1249–1257. https://doi.org/10.1111/cea.13727

9. Poehacker, S., McLaughlin, A., Humiston, T., & Peterson, C. (2021). Assessing parental anxiety in pediatric food allergy: Development of the worry about food allergy questionnaire. *J Clin Psychol Med Settings, 28*(3), 447. https://doi.org/10.1007/s10880-020-09737-1

10. McCuskey Shepley, M. (2005). The health-care environment. In J. A. Rollins, R. Bolig, & C. C. Mahan (Eds.), *Meeting Children's psychosocial needs across the health-care continuum* (pp. 313–349). Pro-ed.

11. Goodyear-Brown, P. (2021). Integrating the therapeutic powers of play in clinical practice settings. In E. Prendiville & J. Parson (Eds.), *Cinical applications of the therapeutic powers of play: Case studies in child and adolescent psychotherapy* (1st ed., pp. 29–45). Routledge.

12. Gordon, J. (2021, 24 February 2021). Emotional safety in pediatrics. Retrieved from https://emotional-safety.org/emotional-safety-in-pediatrics/

13. Staab, J. H., Klayman, G. J., & Lin, L. (2014). Assessing pediatric patient's risk of distress during health-care encounters: The psychometric properties of the psychosocial

risk assessment in pediatrics. *Journal of Child Health Care, 18*(4), 378–387. https://doi.org/10.1177/1367493513496671

14. Levine, P. A., & Kline, M. (2006). *Trauma through a child's eyes: Awakening the ordinary miracle of healing*. North Atlantic Books.

15. Van Der Kolk, B. A. (2014). *The body keeps the score: mind, brain and body in the transformation of trauma*. Penguin books.

16. Forgey, M., & Bursch, B. (2013). Assessment and management of pediatric iatrogenic medical trauma. *Current Psychiatry Reports, 15*(2), 1. https://doi.org/10.1007/s11920-012-0340-5

17. Parson, J. A. (2014). Holistic Mental Health Care & Play Therapy for hospitalised, chronically ill children. In A. Myrick & E. J. Green (Eds.), *Play therapy with vulnerable populations: No child forgotten* (pp. 125–139). Rowman & Littlefield Publishers.

18. McInnes, K. (2019). Being a playful play therapist. In P. Ayling (Ed.), *Becoming and being a play therapist: play therapy in practice* (pp. 99–109). Routledge.

19. Rogers, C. R. (1995). *A way of being*. Mariner Books.

20. Rogers, C. R. (2007). The necessary and sufficient conditions of therapeutic personality change. *Psychotherapy: Theory, Research, Practice, Training, 44*(3), 240–248. https://doi.org/10.1037/0033-3204.44.3.240

21. Olejniczak, K. (2019). The therapeutic dance: the role of affective synchrony in guiding therapists when to lead and when to follow in psychotherapy with traumatized children. In Y. Iorri & G. Ken (Eds.), *Turning points in play therapy and the emergence of self : applications of the play therapy dimensions model* (pp. 187–205). Jessica Kingsley Publishers.

22. Porges, S. (2021). PART ONE the anatomy of calm. *Psychology Today, 54*(5), 36–40.

23. National Institute for the Clinical Application of Behavioral Medicine (NICABM). (2019). How to help your clients understand their window of tolerance. Retrieved from https://www.nicabm.com/trauma-how-to-help-your-clients-understand-their-window-of-tolerance/

24. Gordon, J., & Paisley, S. (2018). Trauma-focused medical play. In L. C. Rubin (Ed.), *Handbook of medical play therapy and child life : interventions in clinical and medical settings* (pp. 154–173). Routledge.

25. Luongo, J., & Vilas, D. B. (2018). Medical makers: therapeutic play using "loose parts". In L. C. Rubin (Ed.), *Handbook of medical play therapy and child life : interventions in clinical and medical settings* (pp. 299–313). Routledge.

26. Cochran, N. H., Cochran, J. L., & Nordling, W. J. (2010). *Child-centered play therapy: A practical guide to developing therapeutic relationships with children*. John Wiley & Sons.

27. Drewes, A. A., & Schaefer, C. E. (2015). The therapeutic powers of play. In L. D. Braverman, K. J. O'Connor, & C. E. Schaefer (Eds.), *Handbook of play therapy* (2nd ed., pp. 35–60). John Wiley & Sons, Inc..

28. Yasenik, L. (2021). Polly meets Maddie: fostering emotional wellness. In E. Prendiville & J. Parson (Eds.), *Clinical applications of the therapeutic powers of play: Case studies in child and adolescent psychotherapy* (1st ed., pp. 29–45). Routledge.

29. Kuttner, L. (2013). The Magic Glove: a Hypnotic Pain Management Technique. Retrieved from https://pediatric-pain.ca/wp-content/uploads/2013/04/The_Magic_Glove12.pdf

30. Baxter, A. L., Cohen, L. L., McElvery, H. L., Lawson, M. L., & von Baeyer, C. L. (2011). An integration of vibration and cold relieves venipuncture pain in a pediatric emergency department. *Pediatric Emergency Care, 27*(12), 1151–1156. https://doi.org/10.1097/PEC.0b013e318237ace4

31. Khanjari, S., Haghani, H., Khoshghadm, M., & Asayesh, H. (2021). The effect of combined external cold and vibration during immunization on pain and anxiety levels in children. *Journal of Nursing & Midwifery Sciences, 8*(4), 231–237. https://doi.org/10.4103/jnms.jnms_128_20

Supporting Evan with Pain

Bridget Sarah

Objectives

At the end of this chapter, you will be able to:

- Explain the presenting medical and developmental issues for children diagnosed with Cerebral Palsy.
- Illustrate the experience of undergoing botulinum toxin injections through the eyes of a child and their family when psychosocial support is limited.
- Present a range of therapeutic interventions and strategies that may protect and heal the emotional self, for children undergoing painful and potentially traumatizing medical procedures.

Introduction

Cerebral Palsy (CP) is the most common physical disability in childhood, with a prevalence rate of one in every 500 live births [1]. It originates from the terms "cerebral" meaning brain, and "palsy" meaning lack of muscle control [2]. CP is characterized by uncontrolled or unpredictable muscle movement, stiffness, weakness, and tightness. Postural and movement symptoms can also be accompanied by breathing, swallowing, communication, intellectual, and digestive difficulties. While children with CP present with a range of abilities, those with significant muscle tightness often experience pain and limited range of movement.

To remediate significant motor impairment, children frequently undergo medical procedures by means of botulinum toxin-A (BOTOX ®) injections to relieve muscle tension and improve movement and comfort. While injections relieve long-term

B. Sarah (✉)
School of Health and Social Development, Deakin University, Geelong, VIC, Australia
e-mail: bridget.sarah@deakin.edu.au

J. A. Parson et al. (eds.), *Integrating Therapeutic Play Into Nursing and Allied Health Practice*, https://doi.org/10.1007/978-3-031-16938-0_12

tightness, remarkable short-term pain and discomfort may be experienced by the child patient, that is not habituated to over repeated treatments. This long-term management is frequently seen to be prioritized over short-term psychosocial health and well-being, with procedures often resulting in traumatic experiences for the child, family, and professionals.

Discourse on the psychosocial iatrogenic trauma for children with CP who undergo these procedures is limited in academic literature. This chapter will take the reader on a journey through the eyes of Evan. Evan is a seven-year-old boy who has experienced Cerebral Palsy which required him to be admitted directly into a regional and then tertiary hospital for specialized treatment including BOTOX © injections. This chapter will consider the world of Evan and his family as they encounter various stages of his treatment.

A therapeutic assessment will be outlined with a range of therapeutic interventions and strategies highlighted in consideration of the health and well-being needs of Evan and his family, as well as the health care professionals tasked with this complex care.

Cerebral Palsy

Cerebral Palsy (CP) is an umbrella term used to diagnose the result of a combination of events either before, during, or after birth that has led to an injury in a baby's developing brain. The condition is a permanent, lifelong physical disability, but it is not unchanging as the individual grows and develops over the lifespan. There is no single cause of CP, with the source remaining unknown for most children. It is accepted that CP arises from a series of causal pathways, i.e., a sequence of events that when combined can cause or accelerate injury to the developing brain, with a small percentage of cases due to complications at birth such as asphyxia [3]. Perinatal stroke, that being focal vascular injury that occurs in the developing brain between 20 weeks of gestation and the 28th postnatal day, is the most common cause of unilateral Cerebral Palsy where damage to major components of the motor system results in lifelong physical disability [4]. In most cases, the brain injury leading to CP is believed to be caused either in utero or before one month of age [5]. Gender differences in CP diagnosis are slight, with a prevalence split of 57 percent of cases being diagnosed in males, and 43 percent in females [5].

Best practice clinical guidelines for the treatment of children with Cerebral Palsy have continued to advance, in step with what is known as "the decade of the brain" from 1990 to 1999 [6] and the mass explosion of neurology research that followed. This led to major advancements in an integrated understanding of brain structure and function. Today, an early, accurate diagnosis of CP is expected, to optimize the principles of neuroplasticity using specific and targeted early intervention [1]. In 2021, the World Health Organizations' Rehabilitation 2030 Initiative convened global content experts to conduct systematic reviews of clinical practice guidelines for 20 chronic health conditions, including Cerebral Palsy. The aim was to develop a set of evidence-based interventions for universal health coverage [7]. The resulting document, titled "Interventions to improve physical function for children and young people with cerebral palsy: International clinical practice guidelines" [8] comprises 13 recommendations for interventions to improve physical function for children and young people with CP.

While the most recent iteration of the international clinical practice guidelines is comprehensive and evidenced by a strong research base, interventions focus primarily on improving physical function for children and young people via approaches such as bimanual therapy and goal-directed training. The guidelines acknowledge that adjunct medical management may be needed for children with severe motor impairment. Recommendation number four states that "Intervention should involve enjoyable, motivating, and challenging activities. If the child is crying or distressed, the clinician should stop, comfort the child, and change the intervention to match the child's needs and preferences. If the intervention is painful and/or distressing, it is not recommended" ([8], pg. 7.). What is absent in the guidelines is psychosocial considerations, or reference to therapeutic interventions and strategies that may complement and enhance the patients' experience of the implementation of these therapies, nor how to protect against the inherent pain and distress caused by medically driven procedures such as BOTOX © injections.

Case Vignette—Evan's Experience

Evan is a 7-year-old boy diagnosed with level four, spastic quadriplegia Cerebral Palsy. This is a bilateral diagnosis, whereby both arms and legs are affected with significant muscle tightness. Children with a level four diagnosis use methods of mobility that require physical or powered assistance, in most settings. Evan is a cheeky young boy, who loves superheroes, electronic games, and outdoor adventure. Evan can walk short distances with the use of ankle foot orthosis and a walking frame. He can play and crawl on the floor when at home and climb onto lounge chairs. He requires physical assistance for transfers, including in and out of the car and on and off the toilet. At school and in the community, Evan uses a manual wheelchair. Evan lives at home with his mother, father, and 10-year-old sister. Evan's mother is his primary carer and assumes most of the responsibility for his day-to-day care, as well as coordination of external supports, such as medical and allied health appointments. As a result of Evans care needs, his mother has reduced her hours of paid work and at times takes substantial amounts of leave away from the workforce. Evans sister frequently assumes caregiving roles assisting Evan with activities of daily living. The demands of caring for Evan have wide-ranging physical, financial, social, and emotional impacts for his family.

In addition to limited mobility, Evan presents with global developmental delay, digestive discomfort due to chronic constipation, and persistent pain. While his pain is managed during the day via engaging activities and periods of rest, Evan's sleep is significantly disrupted due to postural discomfort and unpredictable muscle spasms. For Evan, the continuous cycle of pain and mobility difficulties causes him distress, frustration, fatigue, and a reluctance to try new things. He is hypervigilant to the sensory information in his environment with an increased need for reassurance and predictability to feel safe in all settings. Evan finds it particularly uncomfortable and worrisome to participate in physical therapy.

At the age of three, Evan's care team first recommended the use of botulinum toxin-A (BOTOX ©) injections to reduce muscle overactivity and stiffness, with the aim to reduce pain, improve range of movement and promote general comfort. In the three-to-six-month period following BOTOX ©, patients are required to participate in increased physical therapy with the aim to strengthen their opposing muscles before the temporary effects of BOTOX © wane. While injections relieve longer-term tightness, remarkable short-term pain, and discomfort may be experienced by the child patient, that is not habituated to over repeated treatments [9].

The first time Evan was treated using BOTOX © injections, he and his mother arrived at their local regional rehabilitation center. Neither of them had attended the site before. Evan and his mother were guided to a small clinical room where a range of medical instruments and a plinth bed were located. Evan's mother was reminded of the benefits of BOTOX © treatment and asked to sign a consent form on behalf of her son. She was then instructed to place Evan on the plinth and stand beside him. Evan's mother stroked his forehead and spoke to him about the chocolate frog she had waiting for him in the car when they were finished. The attending doctor applied a topical anesthetic to six sites on Evans' legs, spanning from his groin to calf. Evan was cautious but relaxed and stared up at the imposing male figure above him. The doctor's eyes were friendly, but his mouth and nose were covered with a medical mask, and he was wearing heavy framed glasses. The doctor proceeded to administer the first injection, describing it as "a quick little sting." Evan shrieked in pain, tears sprung to his eyes, and he began flailing his arms and legs attempting to move from the plinth into his mother's arms. "Just a couple more little stings" replied the doctor. A further five injections were administered, with each one Evan becoming increasingly distressed. His mother and an attending nurse each held down one of his arms. A surprisingly heavy amount of force was needed to restrain this small framed and partially immobile boy. At one point, Evan's mother felt herself on the verge of crying. She did not want to show Evan that she too was upset, so she momentarily peered into the nearby wall, taking a few deep breaths to gather herself. Evan searched for her eyes and could not understand why his mother was not helping him. She was sure Evan's screaming would be loud enough to be heard as far as the reception area. Suddenly, the treatment was over. With both Evan and his mum in a state of distress, Evan was carried out to the car, buckled into his car seat and they left. Both Evan and his mother cried the rest of the way home.

In the months that followed, the traumatizing BOTOX © experience was not discussed, and there was no talk or play-based debrief offered for either Evan or his mother. Evan participated in increased clinic-based physical therapy sessions, and his parents implemented new physical therapies into his daily routine. Five months later, the procedure was repeated.

By this time, Evan had celebrated his fourth birthday and had begun preschool. Living in a regional town, Evan's preschool, maternal grandparents house, and the rehabilitation center were all located within a 1-km radius of each other. Evan loved preschool, and while he tired easily, he enjoyed playing in the sandpit and building with the large blocks. Given that he enjoyed going to preschool so much, Evan's mother could not understand why he would begin crying in the car each time they passed through a particular roundabout on their way. After he began displaying the same distress when they would take a similar route to visit his grandparent's house, his mother realized that Evan believed they were on their way to BOTOX © treatment.

As he grew older, and a further two rounds of BOTOX © injections were performed, Evan was becoming increasingly fearful and hypervigilant to the world around him. Evan's mother, having only ever attended the BOTOX © appointments on her own due to her husband's work commitments, felt isolated in the experience and grew resentful toward her husband for having to, in her view, be the parent to inflict such a thing on their child. Evan began refusing to participate in clinic-based physical therapy and would become emotionally distressed at the sight of helping professionals or settings that resembled a clinic like environment, i.e., the general practitioner's office and dentist. To reduce Evan's fears surrounding physical therapy, sessions were offered by visiting professionals in his home. Unfortunately, for Evan, this was experienced as a threatening intrusion into his once predictable, nurturing, and safe space. It was around this time that Evan's care team agreed that his BOTOX © treatment was now outside the scope of the regional setting, and he was referred to a tertiary hospital for specialized treatment.

Psychosocial Iatrogenic Trauma

Discussion on the psychosocial iatrogenic trauma for children with CP who undergo these procedures is limited in academic literature. Similarly, the available therapeutic interventions to prevent, minimize, and resolve the impact on the child's mental health and well-being are often unrecognized, underutilized, or absent within clinical settings and hospitals. Children like Evan with developmentally reduced communication ability and cognitive capacity are particularly vulnerable to perceived cruel treatment and the absence of choice and voice for optimal care preferences. This chapter will now present a summary of the therapeutic assessment of Evan and his family and highlight a range of therapeutic interventions and strategies that may be used to both prevent and ameliorate iatrogenic trauma for children undergoing botulinum toxin injections and their families.

Therapeutic Assessment

Observational assessment, caregiver interview and the "Basic Ph" model of coping and resiliency [10] were utilized to gather information. The "Basic Ph" seeks to understand a person's individual set of coping resources to identify individual preferences and therapeutic approaches to further build resilience. A summary of the assessment outcomes for Evan and his family is as follows.

- Evan was extremely fearful of any setting that resembled a clinical space and all health care professionals. He felt a keen sense of mistrust toward adults with whom he was unfamiliar and was continually uncertain as to whether his parents were the people who would protect and rescue him from painful and scary medical experiences or expose and take part in them against him.
- Evan's nervous system was frequently stuck in a state of hyperarousal and hypervigilance even in the absence of immediate threat or danger. He was increasingly over responsive to sensory information, particularly touch, which was impacting his daily life. For example, Evan could not tolerate grooming tasks such as bathing, haircuts, and nail cutting. He would become dysregulated and lash out at adults when under perceived threat.
- To manage Evan's heightened stress response, his parents had resorted to secret keeping, bribing, and lying about the details of his treatment. Evan's parents were feeling unsure and conflicted about how to help their son access the physical healing that he needed, while questioning if the harm to his emotional being was truly in his best interests. This stress was often a cause of conflict in their marital relationship. Evan's mum reported their confidence as parents reduced "down to zero."
- Evan's sister had become preoccupied with protecting him and following him around the school yard, often complained of tummy aches, and demanded days off from school to stay home and attend appointments with her brother and mother. She would become tearful whenever she was taken to her grandparents to be cared for while Evan went for an outpatient appointment or hospital admission.
- All humans have preferred modes of coping and draw on this in times of stress. The Basic Ph model of coping and resiliency [10] was used to gain an understanding of Evan's temperament, nature, and behavior from the perspective of his individual survival and coping language. Using the Basic Ph, Evan was prompted to draw a six-part story and then tell the story to the therapist. Lahad [10] explains that to tell a projected story based on the elements of fairy tales and myth; we will see the way the child projects themselves in organized reality to meet the world. Fig. 1 shows Evan's six-part story.

Over several years, Evans long-term pain and mobility management had been continually prioritized over short-term psychosocial health and well-being. When a medical experience is perceived by the child as mentally or emotionally overwhelming, this constitutes medical trauma [11]. Vicarious medical trauma is also common in the caregivers and siblings who help to look after them. Levine and Kline [12] explain that medical procedures are by their very nature the most potentially traumatizing to people of all ages due to the feelings of helplessness at the mercy of strangers, in unfamiliar settings while in elevated pain. It is this physical assault to the nervous system that becomes deposited in the emotional memory bank of children. Damaging the emotional being, often an unintended consequence of healing the physical being [13].

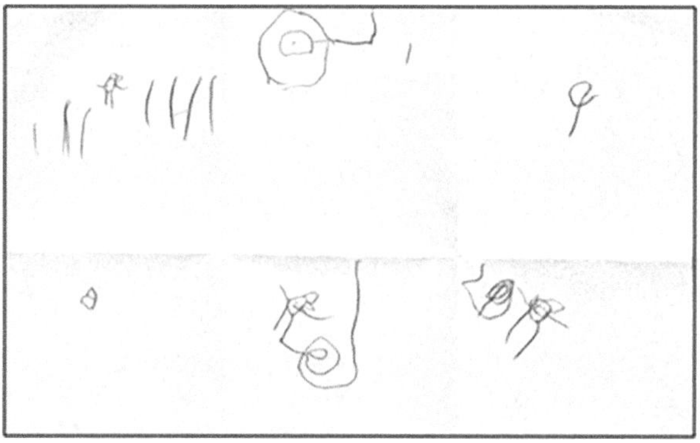

Fig. 1 Evans six-part story as pictured from R–L, top to bottom. There is a flying superhero who lives in the grass (image 1). The superhero is on a mission to remove a stuck key from an electrical outlet (image 2). There is a spare key that would be useful to the superhero (image 3), however, it is locked under padlock (image 4). The superhero uses his kicking strength and "magical strength power" to bust open the padlock (image 5) and thereby freeing the initial key from the electrical outlet (image 6)

Therapeutic Intervention and Play Strategies Tailored for Iatrogenic Trauma

The following section of this chapter will outline a range of practical considerations, provide normative and therapeutic medical play suggestions, as well as consider the systemic supports that may enhance the well-being of Evan's family unit.

Practical Considerations

- Allowing options for physical positioning during procedures is a simple way to return some agency to the child. Comfort positioning is the term used to describe when a caregiver wraps their arms around their child and provides comfort throughout the procedure. Medical and allied health teams should discuss positioning that may work and provide demonstrations to the child, allowing the child to experiment and choose options that they prefer. Allowing caregivers to be a source of support and comfort, rather than discomfort promotes safety and trust in the child–caregiver relationship [14].
- Utilizing the "*Buzzy*" device to combine localized cold and vibration sensory input to reduce needle-related procedural pain [15].

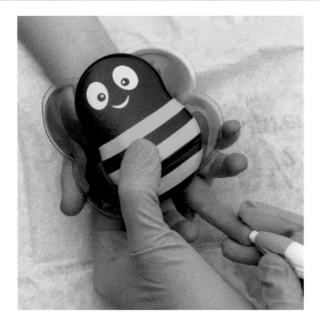

- Distraction methods, requiring either passive or active participation from the patient are an effective method in reducing behavioral responses. Best used from the first treatment, available distraction methods are limitless, based on the child's interests and preference. Nurses, child life therapists, and allied health workers are well placed to use their personal knowledge of their patients to tailor distraction methods [16].
- A felt sense of control over the safe choice of distraction methods may counter against the lack of control felt over medical treatments [17]. Examples include bubbles, puppets, screen time, and immersive technologies such as virtual reality. *Biofeedback-assisted relaxation training* in the form of *heart rate-controlled artworks* to help manage pain and anxiety is of note [18].
- Providing clear and honest explanations and answers to questions, at the child's level of receptive language is core to a felt sense of trust and safety. Photos, picture books, and social stories may support children with less verbal language or lower cognition. It is important to consider the approach-avoidance paradigm where the assumption is that matching interventions with preferred style of coping, i.e., matching distraction with avoidance coping and information provision with attender coping, will result in optimal outcomes during stressful pediatric procedures [19]. Tools such as the Child Approach-Avoidance rating scale [19] and the Behavioral Approach-Avoidance and Distress Scale [20] may be used to supplement observation and parent and medical professional report.

Normative Play

- Frequent opportunities for pediatric patients to engage in normative play is central to emotional wellness. The therapeutic powers of play inherent to normative play, particularly resiliency, positive emotions, stress management, and self-expression will bolster the patients overall coping and well-being. Child Life Therapists and Play Therapists may consider a menu of play experiences tailored for each patient in consideration of their health care needs and the diverse types of play. For example, sensory play to soothe the stress response system, bedside games such as scribble tag and board games where siblings, caregivers, and staff can be involved [21].

Therapeutic and Medical Play

- Medical play in the form of *syringe painting and water play* can be utilized to reduce fear of the medical equipment used to administer BOTOX via familiarization and safe exploration [22].
- Educative medical play, documented with a *procedural support plan*, by a Child Life Therapist or Play Therapist assists to safely prepare the child for an upcoming procedure, reducing anxiety-induced unknowns and thereby enabling acceptance, and participation in care. The use of real-life safe medical equipment is encouraged where possible, as is role play with toys or people and the involvement of trusted others such as siblings and caregivers.
- Post-procedure medical Play Therapy may serve as an opportunity for the child to address complex psychological, emotional, and physical issues resulting from the trauma of BOTOX injections. Post-procedure Play Therapy supports children to communicate their story, express feelings, gain control, and rewrite the endings of their trauma narratives [9].
- Applying assessment findings from the Basic Ph six-part story method [10] can inform prevention and intervention to help the child and family plan for and cope with distressing situations. Where the predominate coping strategy is fixed and rigid, children may benefit from support to expand their tool kit of coping options to gain increased flexibility and capacity in coping with stressful situations.

In the case of Evan, his six-part story demonstrated a preference for utilizing physical activity and the imagination as coping mechanisms. Opportunities for formal and informal physical activity, as well as allocated time for free normative play and arts exploration will encourage self-expression.

Systemic Considerations

- Supportive education for caregivers and siblings may support the general management of the family's mental health care needs at home. Family education regarding physical and emotional medical trauma may be given alongside the formulation of *Behavior Support Profile* that identifies trauma reminders and provides suggested activities for when they do occur.

- Family counselling or psychotherapeutic support, namely Filial Therapy, provided by a qualified Play Therapist may be of benefit. Filial Therapy is a capacity building family based therapy, where parents receive training, supervision, and support as they embark on a process of learning how to conduct therapeutic play sessions with their own children, including siblings. Filial Therapy has an extensive evidence base for improving overall family wellness, functioning, and well-being. Parents report that through Filial Therapy they gain parenting skills and perceive themselves as having an enhanced ability to use their skills to promote positive change in their family [23].

- Compassion fatigue in the form of burnout and secondary trauma is common in health care workers. Staff should have knowledge of recognizing the *signs and symptoms* of compassion fatigue and feel equipped with *self-care and stress management strategies.*

Chapter Summary

Cerebral Palsy is a complex disease where pediatric patients are often required to undergo painful medical procedures in the form of botulinum toxin injections that can cause great distress in the form of iatrogenic trauma. Protecting and healing the emotional self with the same importance as the physical self must become the standard of care. Play therapy professionals should work to advocate for the child's right to psychosocial health and well-being within a system that often priorities physical treatment outcomes. Each health care professional has an integral role in the procedural support team for these children and families, with a range of therapeutic interventions and strategies at their disposal.

Reflective Questions and Activities

- How might you coach a caregiver to hold their 2-year-old child who is coming in for their first botulinum toxin treatment? What comfort positions might they try?
- How might you facilitate normative play at the bedside for a non-ambulatory patient and their sibling during visiting hours?
- Take a moment to visit the clinical space where some procedures are completed in your workplace. Imagine you are a child visiting this space for the first time. What can you see, hear, smell, taste, and touch? Are there changes you can make to this space to promote a felt sense of comfort and safety?
- Discuss some of the ways patients could be introduced to procedures using therapeutic medical play and the language you might use to supplement this.

References

1. Novak, I., Morgan, C., Adde, L., Blackman, J., Boyd, R., Brunstrom, H., Giovanni, C., Damino, D., Darrah, J., Eliasson, A., de Vries, L., Einspieler, C., Fahey, M., Fehlings, D., Ferriero, M., Fetters, L., Fiori, S., et al. (2017). Early, accurate diagnosis and early intervention in cerebral palsy: Advances in diagnosis and treatment. *JAMA Pediatrics, 171*(9), 897–907. https://doi.org/10.1001/jamapediatrics.2017.1689
2. Cerebral Palsy Alliance. (2018). What is Cerebral Palsy? Retrieved from: https://cerebralpalsy.org.au/our-research/about-cerebral-palsy/what-is-cerebral-palsy/.
3. Blair, E. (2010). Epidemiology of the cerebral palsies. *Orthopedics Clinics of North America, 41*(4), 441–455. https://doi.org/10.1016/j.ocl.2010.06.004
4. Woodward, K. E., Carlson, H. L., Kuczynski, A., Saunders, J., Hodge, J., & Kirton, A. (2019). Sensory-motor network functional connectivity in children with unilateral cerebral palsy secondary to perinatal stroke. *NeuroImage: Clinical, 21*, 101670.
5. Australian Cerebral Palsy Register. (2013). Australian Cerebral Palsy Register Report Birth Years 1993–2006.
6. Institute of Medicine (US (United States)). (1991). In C. M. Pechura & J. B. Martin (Eds.), *Committee on a National Neural Circuitry Database. Mapping the brain and its functions: Integrating enabling technologies into neuroscience research.* National Academies Press (US).
7. Damiano, D. L., Longo, E., de Campos, A. C., Forssberg, H., & Rauch, A. (2021). Systematic review of clinical guidelines related to care of individuals with cerebral palsy as part of the World Health Organization efforts to develop a global package of interventions for rehabilitation. *Archives of Physical Medicine and Rehabilitation, 102*(9), 1764–1774.
8. Jackman, M., Sakzewski, L., Morgan, C., Boyd, R. N., Brennan, S. E., Langdon, K., et al. (2021). Interventions to improve physical function for children and young people with cerebral palsy: International clinical practice guideline. *Developmental Medicine & Child Neurology.*
9. Gordon, A., & Paisley, S. (2017). Trauma focused medical play. In L. C. Rubin (Ed.), *Handbook of medical play therapy and child life: Interventions in clinical and medical settings.* Taylor & Francis Group.
10. Lahad, M. (2004). BASIC Ph. The story of coping resources. Retrieved from https://www.espct.eu/fileadmin/espct/documents/articles/BASIC_PhLahadDG.docx
11. Kisiel, C., Lyons, J. S., Blaustein, M., Fehrenbach, T., Griffi, N. G., Germain, J., et al. (2010). *Child and adolescent needs and strengths (CANS) manual: The NCTSN CANS comprehensive—Trauma version: A comprehensive information integration tool for children and adolescents exposed to traumatic events.* Praed Foundation. /Los Angeles, California and Durham, NC: NCTSN.
12. Levine, P. A., & Kline, M. (2006). *Trauma through a child's eyes: Awakening the ordinary miracle of healing.* North Atlantic Books.
13. Parson, J. A. (2014). Holistic mental health care and play therapy for hospitalized chronically ill children. In E. J. Green & A. C. Myrick (Eds.), *Play therapy with vulnerable populations: No child forgotten* (pp. 125–136). Rowman & Littlefield.
14. Royal Childrens Hospital. (2019). Reducing your child's discomfort during procedures. Retrieved from https://www.rch.org.au/Reduce_childrens_discomfort_during_procedures/
15. Ballard, A., Khadra, C., Adler, S., Trottier, E. D., & Le May, S. (2019). Efficacy of the buzzy device for pain management during needle-related procedures. *The Clinical Journal of Pain, 35*(6), 532–543.
16. Drape, K., & Greenshields, S. (2020). Using play as a distraction technique for children undergoing medical procedures. *British Journal of Nursing, 29*(3), 142–143.
17. Koller, D., & Goldman, R. D. (2012). Distraction techniques for children undergoing procedures: A critical review of pediatric research. *Journal of Pediatric Nursing, 27*(6), 652–681.
18. Khut, G., Morrow, A., Yogui-Watanabe, M. (2011). The BrightHearts Project: A new approach to the management of procedure-related paediatric anxiety. Retrieved from https://www.georgekhut.com/

19. Bernard, R. S., Cohen, L. L., McClellan, C. B., & MacLaren, J. E. (2004). Pediatric procedural approach-avoidance coping and distress: A multitrait-multimethod analysis. *Journal of Pediatric Psychology, 29*(2), 131–141.
20. Hubert, N. C., Jay, S. M., Saltoun, M., & Hayes, M. (1988). Approach—avoidance and distress in children undergoing preparation for painful medical procedures. *Journal of Clinical Child Psychology*, 17(3), 194–202.
21. Burns-Nader, S., & Hernandez-Reif, M. (2016). Facilitating play for hospitalized children through child life services. *Children's Health Care, 45*(1), 1–21. https://doi.org/10.108 0/02739615.2014.948161
22. Malchiodi, C. A., & Goldring, E. (2012). Art therapy and child life. *Art Therapy and Health Care, 48*.
23. Cornett, N., & Bratton, S. C. (2015). A golden intervention: 50 years of research on filial therapy. *International Journal of Play Therapy, 24*(3), 119.

Connor Struggles to Stay in School

Kate L. Renshaw

Objectives

At the end of this chapter, you will be able to:

- Develop an initial understanding of how early life trauma can influence bio-psycho-social health and child development.
- Review suitable assessments for paediatric mental health practice at the intersection site of both health and education services.
- Consider a case example that aims to bring to life a complex case involving medical, education, and psychotherapeutic service provisions in a community-based setting.
- Reflect on three self-care resources targeted at preventing and countering secondary traumatic stress and compassion fatigue.

Introduction

Play Therapy is a long-established psychotherapeutic modality for working with children in diverse settings such as clinical, educative, and community based [1]. Meta-analyses indicated that Play Therapy is developmentally and culturally sensitive across a broad range of presenting paediatric mental health difficulties, with a beneficial treatment effect [2, 3]. Humanistic models of Play Therapy that include parents produce the most beneficial treatment outcomes [3]. This chapter is based on a composite case example that details a systemic Play Therapy approach to support the child, Connor, in a developmentally sensitive manner.

K. L. Renshaw (✉)
School of Health and Social Development, Deakin University, Geelong, VIC, Australia
e-mail: kate.renshaw@deakin.edu.au

J. A. Parson et al. (eds.), *Integrating Therapeutic Play Into Nursing and Allied Health Practice*, https://doi.org/10.1007/978-3-031-16938-0_13

Meeting Connor in the Clinical Setting

Connor's eyes were closed. He could feel the chilly wind on his face; it was bitterly cold. He could hear the muffled sounds of other children playing in the playground. He did not really want to be here, and he thought about what mum would be doing right now at home. Then, he heard the school bell ring. His eyes snapped open. He was immediately running towards the door that connected the playground to the classroom. He did not want to be late! His teacher greeted him at the door; he knelt and said quietly, *"Mum is here to see you, go meet her at our classroom door"*. He was excited as he was just thinking about mum, but then he wondered to himself, *"what mum is doing here... it's only the end of morning playtime?"* He saw mum and started running towards her. She smiled and scooped him up into a hug. He melted into her hug; it was so good to see her! She said, *"Did you remember, we are meeting Kate today...the Play Therapist in school?"* Connor had forgotten about this; he shook his head side to side letting mum know he had not remembered. Mum held his hand and they walked together through the school's corridors and into the connecting community centre. It smelt different in the community centre to the school. He had always liked it there as he had come to the community centre with mum before for things like playgroup and day care. He thought it smelt like biscuits and warm milk. Connor asked mum, *"Is this where we are going to see Kate?"* Mum said it was where she had her playroom and children and families from school came to see her there. He was relieved, as he liked the community centre. Connor was also a bit curious to see who Kate was, in case he had seen her around school before. Mum knocked on the door at the end of the corridor. The door opened and he saw Kate. He watched her for a few moments as she introduced herself, she seemed friendly. As she welcomed them into the room, he realised she *was* familiar, he had seen her around school. His body relaxed a little as he sat down in a chair next to mum. He looked around the room; there was a lot to see, he was a bit overwhelmed, he held mum's hand and waited to see when he could play with the toys.

Background to the Presenting Condition

The School Nurse (SN), who is a Specialist Community Public Health Nurse, referred Connor and his mother, Gerry, to the *British Association of Play Therapists* (BAPT) Registered Play Therapist®. Referral information included the history of both family and school concerns in relation to Connor's difficulties with incontinence (enuresis and encopresis). The SN had previously supported Gerry to explore Connor's continence difficulties with both his General Practitioner (GP) and subsequently a hospital referral to a multi-disciplinary paediatric specialist clinic at the children's hospital in their region. The hospital clinic assessed Connor's incontinence and concluded that there was no underlying physical reason for this and recommended that Connor and his mother receive continence education and therapeutic support. The therapeutic support rationale was based on the history of Family Violence (FV) as reported by Connor's mother. The SN and Gerry discussed a range of options for Connor to access psychological services and decided on accessing the service provided by the school Play Therapist.

Literature on the Presenting Condition

The supporting literature for the psychotherapy modality of Play Therapy aligns with the reasons for referral including family violence [4–6], developmental trauma [7–9], and attachment difficulties [10–13]. As elimination disorders were the primary focus for the referral to Play Therapy, a summary of the supporting literature is detailed.

Elimination Disorders

Encopresis and Enuresis are both categorised as Elimination Disorders in both the American Psychiatric Association's Diagnostic and Statistical Manual of Mental Disorders (DSM–5) and the *International Classification of Diseases 11th Revision* (ICD-11). The ICD-11 defines Elimination Disorders as "the repeated voiding of urine into clothes or bed (enuresis) and the repeated passage of faeces in inappropriate places (encopresis)" ([14], para. 2). It is advised that elimination disorders should only be considered after the age of expected continence (4 years for encopresis and 5 years for enuresis).

Play Therapy-specific literature on elimination disorders inclusive of encopresis and enuresis is scant, with only four Play Therapy publications mentioning encopresis and/or enuresis. Enuresis was first mentioned in the Play Therapy literature in 1982 [15]. The case study presented by Noll and Seagull [15] recommended a child-centred therapeutic approach that integrated behavioural and Play Therapy modalities. The paper considered the child's sense of autonomy, mastery, and control as central in the treatment plan for enuresis. Secondly, Knell and Moore [16] published a case study on cognitive-behavioural Play Therapy for encopresis. In this case example, a parent-implemented behaviour management programme was combined with individual cognitive-behavioural Play Therapy, and outcomes were reported for the cessation of encopresis. Thirdly, a case study using child-centred Play Therapy to treat encopresis and enuresis differed from the previous behavioural and cognitive-behavioural publications [17]. In this case study the child

> was able to resolve his underlying fears, doubts, and frustrations in a safe environment, which resulted in his choice to change his behaviour... increased his self-awareness, allowing for further growth in self-esteem and self-actualization... [and] was able to explore and master his environment without feelings of anxiety about being judged or ridiculed. (p. 224)

As a result, Child-Centred Play Therapy (CCPT) facilitated the attainment of continence. It is important to note that the author suggested that an integrative approach to treatment could be considered by clinicians when working with this population [17]. The fourth and final publication only included brief description of cases which included elimination disorders as part of a broader survey of Filipino Play Therapists [18].

Two other publications of interest emerged. The first, researched in Argentina, included a medical publication on play with clay as a therapeutic treatment approach for six children aged 4–12 years [19]. This publication noted that "modelling clay... is a good method of expression for severely constipated children who are still relatively poor at expressing themselves with words" ([19], p. 487). The other publications included a biobehavioural approach that detailed a treatment plan for encopresis in children [20]. The treatment phases of this biobehavioural approach may be useful to note for integrative therapeutic treatment. The phases included demystification, bowel evacuation, toileting schedule, monitoring, feedback, cleanliness training, dietary changes, facilitating medication, and fading facilitative medication [20]. The lack of literature on the presenting condition provided a starting point to commence clinical case conceptualisation with Connor.

Case Conceptualisation

The play therapist's clinical experience and knowledge, together with the referral information for Connor, informed the case conceptualisation process. All previous assessment and diagnostic information were included with the Play Therapy referral. Information included past assessments and recommendations from the General Practitioner (GP), the multi-disciplinary paediatric specialist clinic at the children's hospital, and the SN. The SN provided access to relevant medical history, assessments, diagnoses, and reports. Because the Play Therapist was employed at the school, they had access to Connor's education records, inclusive of assessments, academic reports, and teacher perceptions on overall functioning.

Medical, Connor's continence difficulties had been identified as an elimination disorder with the recommendation for continence education and psychotherapeutic support. The Play Therapist had previous experience with continence difficulties and held knowledge of psychosocial development in childhood.

Educational, Connor had been identified as an anxious school refuser who presented with separation anxiety. As the Play Therapist worked in an education setting, anxiety connected with school attendance and separation from caregivers was familiar with clinical casework.

Psychosocial, the Play Therapist was cognisant of the impact of Connor's experience of family violence and therefore an attachment and developmental trauma lens informed the case conceptualisation.

Integration of medical, educational, and psychosocial aspects of the intake process informed the case planning prior to commencing work with Connor as well as ongoing clinical reasoning.

Individualised Intervention Design

Connor's individualised therapeutic intervention consisted of four phases:

1. Therapeutic Assessment [21, 22].
2. Humanistic Play Therapy (HPT) [23].
3. Individual family Filial Therapy [21, 24].
4. School-based Professional Development (PD) workshop.

Firstly, the therapeutic assessment phase consisted of an assessment session and three individual HPT sessions. The assessment phase allowed the Play Therapist to get to know Connor, Gerry, and the wider system of support, as well as gauge the suitability of HPT as a therapeutic modality and the commitment of the family and system of support for systemic family work. After the three initial HPT sessions, Connor was offered a further 12 HPT sessions with two review meetings after sessions 5 and 11. The second review meeting included planning for the transition to the next phase of the intervention. A 12-session Filial Therapy phase enabled the Play Therapist to support Gerry to learn some therapeutic skills from Play Therapy to use with Connor during supported "special play times" [24] (see Chap. 1 for definitions of Play Therapy and Filial Therapy). The final step in the therapeutic intervention was a Professional Development (PD) workshop for the school staff, which included Connor's educational team and the SN.

Considerations for Health Care Needs Based on Diagnosis

The multi-disciplinary paediatric specialist hospital clinic had considered Connor's exposure to trauma from family violence when diagnosing and providing treatment recommendations. This aligned with the holistic health and wellbeing approach of the Play Therapist and Connor's school. The Play Therapist worked closely with Gerry and the SN to ensure the recommendation for continence education was integrated into Connor's therapeutic treatment plan. The Play Therapist reviewed the educative materials and made recommendations on ensuring a playful approach was taken with Connor concerning continence education. The "Poop it kit" (see Chap. 3) is an example of a playful and creative way to learn about bowel function. Psychoeducation was provided by the Play Therapist to both the SN and Gerry in relation to children's physical and emotional regulation and their "window of tolerance" for the continence education to be informed by Connor's state of arousal [25]. When a child is within their window of optimal arousal, they are better able to notice and cope with both physical and emotional regulation [25]. Please refer to the "Additional resources" section in this chapter for links to the resources recommended in this section.

The Assessment Phase

A detailed referral from the SN, alongside the intake meeting between the Play therapist and Gerry, facilitated the selection of suitable assessment tools and allowed the Play Therapist to get to know Connor [21]. Several questionnaires were selected to contextualise Gerry's early life experiences, including the Adverse Childhood Experiences (ACEs) and Playtime exercise. The Paediatric ACEs and Related Life Events Screener (PEARLS) questionnaire was chosen to screen for adversity in Connor's life. Additionally, the Strength and Difficulties Questionnaires (SDQ) was chosen to monitor change before and after the intervention. Finally, three projective creative arts assessments were selected to assist the Play Therapist to learn more about Connor's emotional state (Blob tree), sense of attachment (3D Birds nest), and family composition and dynamics (Family play genogram). These projective assessments can also be incorporated into post-assessment to track therapeutic progress.

Adverse Childhood Experiences

Firstly, due to the history of family violence, a parental Adverse Childhood Experiences (ACEs) screening questionnaire was conducted (https://www.ace-saware.org/learn-about-screening/screening-tools/). Gerry was provided the choice between an identifiable or de-identified ACEs questionnaire, and she indicated she was comfortable identifying her ACEs. Gerry's ACEs score was a 6/10, indicating that she was in the higher risk category. See additional resources section on administration and scoring of ACEs.

Playtime Exercise

To learn more about Gerry's own childhood play experiences, the Play Therapy Dimensions Model (PTDM) Appendix D—Playtime Exercise was completed [26]. This showed the limited opportunities and resources for play that Gerry was afforded as a child and the absence of a caregiver's presence within the play. During the ACEs questionnaire, she indicated that her teachers and school had really looked out for her, and she mentioned the opportunities within relationships for play she had at primary school. Identifying this Positive Childhood Experience (PCE) was important and informed the therapeutic intervention [27].

Paediatric ACEs and Related Life Events Screener

With Gerry's raised ACEs score in mind, the Paediatric ACEs and Related Life Events Screener (PEARLS) was then completed by Gerry for Connor (https://www.acesaware.org/wp-content/uploads/2019/12/PEARLS-Tool-Child-Parent-Caregiver-

Report-De-Identified-English.pdf). Connor's PEARLS score in part one was 7/10 (the higher risk category) and in part two 2/7, indicating adversity in two areas of Social Determinants of Health (SDOH). See additional resources section on administration and scoring of PEARLS.

Strength and Difficulties Questionnaires

To learn more about Connor's bio-psycho-social functioning, a Strength and Difficulties Questionnaire (SDQ) was completed by Gerry and his teacher (https:// www.sdqinfo.org/a0.html) [28]. Parent and Teacher SDQ scores indicated that Connor was experiencing difficulties across all domains (emotional, conduct, hyperactivity, externalising, internalising, prosocial, and total difficulties) that ranged from slightly raised to very high.

Getting to Know Connor through Projective Assessments

After his initial meeting with Kate and prior to Connor's first Play Therapy session, he attended a play-based assessment session where he completed a series of projective creative arts assessments [29]. The assessments were carefully selected to form a developmentally appropriate method of getting to know Connor prior to the Play Therapy sessions. Throughout this assessment session, the Play Therapist (referred to as Kate in the case exemplars below) made therapeutic verbal and non-verbal responses which facilitated Connor's emotional expression and supported the developing therapeutic relationship [30, 31].

Blob Tree

To start the session, Kate asked Connor to look at the Blob Tree picture [32] and choose and colour (from a range of coloured pencils provided) the blob that represented him. He pointed to a blob lying on the ground, not close to other blobs or the tree, arms crossed in front with a downturned mouth and eyebrows. As he coloured it with a blue pencil, he said, "this blob looks like me today at lunchtime. I was by myself. I was a bit mad because it was cold, and I didn't want to be outside. I wanted to be home with mum; it's warm there".

3D Birds Nest

Next, Connor was invited to use the available arts and craft materials to "create a birds nest", a three-dimensional version of the Birds Nest Drawing (BND) [30]. He got to work straight away and spoke quietly as he created. First, he scanned the available resources and chose the ball of natural twine, scissors, and glue. He then cut many short pieces of twine into a pile. He chose an A4 piece of yellow paper and then used the glue stick in spiral motions on the centre of the page. The cut pieces of twine were then arranged haphazardly on the glued section of the page; he completed this step very quickly and was quiet as he worked. To finish, he selected two pom-pom balls, one big and one small. They were both orange. The two pom-poms were glued in the centre of the twine nest; they were glued right next to each other. During this crafting time, Connor had initially spoken about what he had been doing that day at school, but his conversation quickly turned to talk of his mother and the things they do together. Most of his stories involved time spent with his mother at home.

Family Play Genogram

Finally, Connor was invited to create a family play genogram [33, 34]. The therapist placed an A3 piece of paper with hand-drawn concentric circles from the edge of the paper into the centre (see Fig. 1). Connor was then invited to "show [his] thoughts and feelings about everyone in their family, including [him]" and any other significant people in his life ([33], p. 5). He was invited to choose small toy miniature figurines for each person (from a wide range of symbols) and place them wherever he wanted on the paper. Connor explored the categorised trays of miniature figurines. He selected a figurine quickly, a chimpanzee adult cradling a smaller chimpanzee. It was one figure, with both chimpanzees connected. He placed it in the centre of the page, as indicated by the cross in Fig. 1. Connor was quiet; a narrative did not naturally accompany his genogram. The Play Therapist used several prompts (adapted from [34], p. 56); the questions and answers were:

Q. Could you tell me about this small toy?
A. "It's me and mum".
Q. What might this toy say if it could speak?
A. "We are hanging out at home together".
Q. I wonder what this toy is feeling or thinking.
A. "They're happy".

Fig. 1 Family play genogram using concentric circles

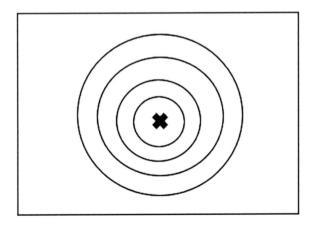

Connor's Play Therapy

Connor hunched over his piece of paper at the table in the playroom. He wore a smock that covered his arms and body. Kate, his play therapist, sat next to him on a small chair, the same size as Connor's. He was immersed in his finger painting. Using different fingers, he transferred assorted colours from the paint palette onto the white A3-sized paper. He then moved his fingers and hands around the page, smearing the colours together. Kate spoke quietly as Connor worked in silence. She observed his actions and narrated what she could see him doing in the play— *"putting red on your pointer finger...placing it on the paper and moving it around... the page is filling up with different paint colours...your hands are mixing...swirling together...the colours are changing..."*. After several minutes of repeating this play, the page was filled with swirls of brown. Connor asked if he could wash his hands. Kate had a bowl of warm soapy water next to the table and a soft hand towel ready. Connor again spent several minutes cleaning his hands, he moved his hands in the water and rubbed them together, the colour of the water started to change. Kate had moved with him and was crouched beside him close to the bowl holding onto the towel. Again, she used verbal reflections as Connor washed—*"your hands are going into the water, maybe it is a little warm...touching the bubbles...swaying your hands in the water...the colour is starting to wash off...rubbing your hands together, your hands might feel a bit slimy..."*. He then asked Kate to dry his hands. Kate engaged with Connor and verbalised what they were doing—*"you're placing your hands on the fluffy towel...I'm using my hands to put pressure on your hands through the towel...working together to dry all over your hands..."*. As Connor worked with Kate to dry his hands, they were standing face to face; Kate had crouched onto her knees to be at the same height as Connor. Every so often Connor would look into Kate's eyes and smile before returning to watching his hands being dried.

This mess-making and hand-washing play sequence occurred in all of Connor's play sessions and was often repeated multiple times within sessions. Towards the end of his play sessions, the finger painting ceased, and he painted with brushes. Painting with brushes allowed him to explore the changing colours of the jar of water as he rinsed his brush between colours. The exploratory sensory play that occurred in every play session at times included other sensory resources such as play dough, clay, and brown "toilet noise putty" that was housed in a toilet-shaped container.

Systemic Practice

Throughout the therapy, a holistic person-centred and systemically focused intervention included the child, family, Play Therapist, educators, and medical professionals. A critical component was timely feedback to medical professionals (namely SN and GP) at the completion of each of the three phases of the intervention. In addition, regular consultation with school staff included targeted feedback and recommendations to assist the educators to support Connor's bio-psycho-social development and wellbeing in school.

Reflection on the Case Conceptualisation Process

Any referral to a Play Therapist benefits from a thorough intake meeting with the parent/s to discuss the life history of the child, from point of conception to present day. This was especially important for the work with Connor and Gerry as family violence had been prevalent during the time of his conception and during his early years of development. The intake meeting was also a valuable time to commence therapeutic alliance building with Gerry. As a survivor of family violence, this process needed to be slow and careful, building trust gradually through consistent therapeutic messages. Therapeutic skills were carefully implemented so that the referral information could be acquired without risk of re-traumatisation. Due to the complexity of the case, a therapeutic assessment was initially identified as the most suitable start to therapeutic work. As Connor engaged well with the initial Play Therapy sessions in the therapeutic assessment phase, a medium-term individual intervention and filial therapy intervention were deemed suitable; the four-phased intervention consisted of approximately 30 contact sessions.

Reasons for referral can feed-forward into the selection of suitable toys and expressive resources ahead of a therapeutic intervention. For Connor, this included toy and resource considerations for encopresis and enuresis exploration in the playroom. Ensuring that embodiment play [35, 36], and messy/sensory play [37, 38] resources were available was therefore particularly important. These included: finger-paints, clay (darker earth brown tone), play-doh® (a variety of colours including brown), slime, and toilet noise putty. Projective play resources were also an important consideration; these included a doll's house with a toilet that had movable parts and human figures with articulated joints or bendable and projective art and craft materials [23]. Finally, early relational play toys and resources to support attachment play [23] were key, these included: a pop-up tent and tunnel, scarves, and larger fabric pieces (suitable for peek-a-boo and hiding), a blanket, baby dolls and toys to care for a baby, a medical kit, bubbles to blow, puppets, and board games such as Jenga® and Connect Four®.

In summary, the case example of Connor has allowed for an examination of medical, education, and psychotherapeutic services working collaboratively. The SN, in this case, facilitated a community-based therapeutic service, which was in line with medical and education recommendations and most importantly was the choice of the parent for her child. The Play Therapist, with consent from Gerry and assent from Connor, shared pertinent feedback and recommendations throughout the intervention to support the family systemically in both the medical and educative domains.

Connor's Play Therapy intervention ameliorated the impact of past trauma on his development. His toileting difficulties reduced and his school attendance increased; cessation of the elimination disorder and attendance within average parameters were achieved by the time of the discharge phase in Filial Therapy.

Reflective Resources and Activities

When working with complex cases, it is wise for the professionals involved to incorporate trauma-informed professional practice activities to care for the self and protect against secondary traumatic stress and compassion fatigue [39]. In this section, three reflective resources and aligned activities utilized by the Play Therapist are detailed below under the following headings: titration and reciprocal inhibition, reflective journaling, and self-care.

Titration and Reciprocal Inhibition

Titration and reciprocal inhibition can be used as a method of reducing the impact of secondary traumatic stress and compassion fatigue. "Titration is based on the notion that exposure to traumatic material is measured and engaged…in small manageable 'doses' and then returning to a sense of resourcing or grounding before returning to the traumatic material" ([40], p. 269). And "Reciprocal inhibition is based on the notion that the relaxation response, which involves decreased levels of psychological and physiological arousal, is antithetical to the trauma response, which involves anxiety and increased levels of physiological arousal" ([40], p. 269). Both titration and reciprocal inhibition are useful tools for health and mental health clinicians. Titration in clinical practice may include considering your daily workflow when working on complex cases to allow for breaks and moments of titration between complex cases. Reciprocal inhibition resources can also be used to either titrate exposure or pair with exposure to traumatic content. Easily accessible reciprocal inhibition resources include breath work and access to nature. In Malchiodi's [41] "Appendix 4. Breathing Prompts" (p.373), examples include foursquare breathing, star breathing, and figure-eight breathing, which provide an array of choice for breath work. Further reading around accessing nature as a resource can be useful [42, 43]. When reviewing literature on nature, consider keywords and concepts such as awe, forest bathing, and blue mind theory [44, 45].

Reflective Journaling

Reflective journaling in the form of written and/or creative arts journaling is a useful resource that many mental health clinicians experience as part of their training [46]. Clinicians who have learnt reflective journaling when training often go on to use it as a resource when practising. If you are not familiar with reflective journaling, consider reviewing literature on both written and creative arts journaling and trialling it yourself.

Self-Care

Developing and maintaining robust self-care practices when practising as a health or mental health clinician are important considerations. Self-care is vital as a career-long practice. Developing and maintaining individualised self-care practices could be considered and monitored within management and/or clinical supervision. For ideas on developing an individualised self-care kit, see the additional resources section below [47].

Additional Resources

- ACEs Aware Clinical Team Toolkit: Preventing, Screening, and Responding to the impact of ACEs and toxic stress. https://www.acesaware.org/wp-content/uploads/2020/05/ACEs-Aware-Provider-Toolkit-5.21.20.pdf
- For continence-related information and resources for children, families, healthcare workers, and educators, refer to ERIC, the Children's Bowel and Bladder Charity website. https://www.eric.org.uk/
- The Bristol Stool Chart can be useful for psychoeducation with children and families. Some families choose to hang this chart on the back of the toilet door and use the various categories to dialogue together. A downloadable/printable JPEG is available at https://pediatricsurgery.stanford.edu/Conditions/BowelManagement/bristol-stool-form-scale.html
- Like the Bristol Stool Chart, the Am I drinking enough water? Urine colour chart can also be useful for psychoeducation with children and families. Some families choose to hang this chart on the back of the toilet door and use the distinct categories to dialogue together. A downloadable/printable PDF is available at http://media.healthdirect.org.au/publications/Urine-Colour-Chart.pdf
- Continence advice often includes elevating the legs to assist in full elimination of faeces and urine. Either a small stool or a specifically designed product such as the Squattypotty® (https://www.squattypotty.com/) can be a useful resource to assist the whole family with complete and successful elimination. Parents and children dialoguing in a normative and matter-of-fact manner around healthy elimination practices can be a useful inclusion for psychoeducation.
- Sensory play ideas are a useful recommendation to families and educators for children who have experienced both developmental trauma and continence difficulties. Access some sensory play ideas here https://www.healthline.com/health/childrens-health/sensory-play#takeaway.
- A visual aide for the Window of Tolerance. https://www.nicabm.com/trauma-how-to-help-your-clients-understand-their-window-of-tolerance/.
- The Self-Care Starter Kit is a freely accessible online resource to support clinicians to develop their own self-care plan, as well as accessing to self-care assessments, exercises, and activities [47]. Begin your self-care journey or continue it using this self-care kit. http://www.socialwork.buffalo.edu/students/self-care/index.asp

References

1. Axline, V. M. (1969). *Play therapy*. Ballantine Books.
2. Bratton, S. C., & Lin, Y. (2015). A meta-analytic review of child-centered play therapy approaches. *Journal of Counseling & Development, 93*, 45–58.
3. Bratton, S. C., Ray, D., Rhine, T., & Jones, L. (2005). The efficacy of play therapy with children: A meta-analytic review of treatment outcomes. *Professional Psychology, Research And Practice, 4*, 376.
4. Brooke, S. L. (2008). *The use of the creative therapies with survivors of domestic violence*. Charles C Thomas Publisher.
5. Hall, J. G. (2019). Child-centered play therapy as a means of healing children exposed to domestic violence. *International Journal of Play Therapy, 28*(2), 98–106.
6. Woollett, N., Bandeira, M., & Hatcher, A. (2020). Trauma-informed art and play therapy: Pilot study outcomes for children and mothers in domestic violence shelters in the United States and South Africa. *Child Abuse & Neglect, 107*.
7. Barfield, S., Dobson, C., Gaskill, R., & Perry, B. D. (2012). Neurosequential model of therapeutics in a therapeutic preschool: Implications for work with children with complex neuropsychiatric problems. *International Journal of Play Therapy, 21*(1), 30–44.
8. Goodyear-Brown, P. (2019). *Trauma and play therapy: Helping children heal*. Routledge.
9. Perry, B. (2014). The neurosequential model of therapeutics. In K. Brandt, B. D. Perry, S. Seligman, & E. Tronick (Eds.), *Infant and early childhood mental health: Core concepts and clinical practice: Vol. first edition* (pp. 21–54). American Psychiatric Association Publishing.
10. Courtney, J. A. (2020). *Infant play therapy: Foundations, models, programs, and practice*. Routledge.
11. Malchiodi, C. A., & Crenshaw, D. A. (2013). *Creative arts and play therapy for attachment problems*. Guilford Publications.
12. Mellenthin, C. (2019). *Attachment centered play therapy*. Routledge.
13. Spooner, M. C. (2020). *Attachment-focused family play therapy. An Intervention for Children and Adolescents after Trauma*. Routledge.
14. ICD-11 (2022, February). ICD-11 for mortality and morbidity statistics. Elimination disorders. Retrieved from https://icd.who.int/browse11/l-m/en#/http://id.who.int/icd/entity/1884115764
15. Noll, R. B., & Seagull, A. A. (1982). Beyond informed consent: Ethical and philosophical considerations in using behavior modification or play therapy in the treatment of enuresis. *Journal of Clinical Child Psychology, 11*(1), 44.
16. Knell, S. M., & Moore, D. J. (1990). Cognitive-Behavioral play therapy in the treatment of encopresis. *Journal of Clinical Child Psychology, 19*(1), 55.
17. Cuddy-Casey, M. (1997). A case study using child-centered play therapy approach to treat enuresis and encopresis. *Elementary School Guidance & Counseling, 31*(3), 220–225.
18. Trivino-Dey, M. L., Dela Paz-Catipon, M. A. A., Tarroja, M. C. H., & Garcia, W. C. C. (2017). Play therapy in the Philippines. In A. F. Y. Siu & A. K. L. Pon (Eds.), *Play therapy in Asia* (pp. 153–172). The Chinese University of Hong Kong Press.
19. Feldman, P. C., Villanueva, S., Lanne, V., & Devroede, G. (1993). Use of play with clay to treat children with intractable encopresis. *The Journal of Pediatrics, 122*(3), 483–488.
20. Friman, P. C., Hofstadter, K. L., & Jones, K. M. (2006). A biobehavioral approach to the treatment of functional encopresis in children. *Journal of Early and Intensive Behavior Intervention, 3*(3), 263–272.
21. Renshaw, K., & Parson, J. (2020). Infant filial therapy – From conception to early years. In J. A. Courtney (Ed.), *Infant play therapy: Foundations, models, programs and practice* (pp. 101–116). Routledge.
22. Ryan, V., & Wilson, K. (2000). *Case studies in non-directive play therapy*. Jessica Kingsley Publishers.

23. Renshaw, K. L., & Parson, J. A. (2021). It's a small world: Projective play. In E. Prendiville & J. Parson (Eds.), *Clinical applications of the therapeutic powers of play: Case studies in child and adolescent psychotherapy* (pp. 72–86). Routledge.
24. VanFleet, R. (2005). *Filial therapy: Strengthening parent-child relationships through play* (2nd ed.). Sarasota, Florida: Professional Resource Press.
25. Siegel, D. J. (2020). *The developing mind: How relationships and the brain interact to shape who we are* (3rd ed.). The Guilford Press.
26. Yasenik, L., & Gardner, K. (2012). *Play therapy dimensions model: A decision-making guide for integrative play therapists* (2nd ed.). Jessica Kingsley Publishers.
27. Bethell, C., Jones, J., Gombojav, N., Linkenbach, J., Sege, R. (2019). Positive Childhood experiences and adult mental and relational health in a Statewide sample: Associations across adverse childhood experiences levels. JAMA Pediatrics. Retrieved from https://jamanetwork.com/journals/jamapediatrics/fullarticle/2749336.
28. Goodman, R. (1997). The strengths and difficulties questionnaire: A research note. *Journal of Child Psychology and Psychiatry, 38*(5), 581–586.
29. Malchiodi, C. A. (1998). *Understanding children's drawings*. Guilford Press.
30. Malchiodi, C. A. (2013). Art therapy, attachment, and parent-child dyads. In C. A. Malchiodi & D. A. Crenshaw (Eds.), *Creative arts and play therapy for attachment problems* (pp. 52–66). Guilford Publications.
31. Schaefer, C. E., & Drewes, A. A. (2014). *The therapeutic powers of play: 20 core agents of change* (2nd ed.). John Wiley & Sons.
32. Wilson, P., & Long, I. (2018). *The big book of blob trees* (2nd ed.). Routledge.
33. Gil, E., & Drewes, A. A. (Eds.). (2021). *Cultural issues in play therapy* (2nd ed.). Guilford Publications.
34. Steele, W., & Malchiodi, C. A. (2012). *Trauma-informed practices with children and adolescents*. Routledge.
35. Jennings, S. (1999). *Introduction to developmental playtherapy: Playing and health*. Jessica Kingsley.
36. Jennings, S., Gerhardt, C., & Ebooks Corporation. (2011). *Healthy attachments and neurodramatic-play*. Jessica Kingsley Publishers.
37. Prendiville, S. (2021a). Sensory play therapy. In H. Kaduson & C. E. Schaefer (Eds.), *Play therapy with children: Modalities for change* (pp. 157–176). American Psychological Association.
38. Prendiville, S. (2021b). Calming Christopher. In E. Prendiville & J. Parson (Eds.), *Clinical applications of the therapeutic powers of play: Case studies in child and adolescent psychotherapy* (pp. 59–71). Routledge.
39. Carello, J., & Butler, L. D. (2015). Practicing what we teach: Trauma-informed educational practice. *Journal of Teaching in Social Work, 35*(3), 262–268.
40. Black, T. G. (2006). Teaching trauma without traumatizing: Principles of trauma treatment in the training of graduate counselors. *Traumatology, 12*(4), 266–271.
41. Malchiodi, C. A. (2020). *Trauma and expressive arts therapy: Brain, body, and imagination in the healing process*. The Guilford Press.
42. Chown, A. (2014). *Play therapy in the outdoors: Taking play therapy out of the playroom and into natural environments*. Jessica Kingsley Publishers.
43. Louv, R. (2016). *Vitamin N: The essential guide to a nature-rich life*. Atlantic Books.
44. Filstrup, C. T. (2019). Blue mind: The surprising science that shows how being near, in, on, or under water can make you happier, healthier, more connected, and better at what you do. *Limnology & Oceanography Bulletin, 28*(3), 114.
45. Livneh, Y. (2015). *Rising on water: play therapy in a new form*. Createspace Independent Publishing Platform.
46. Malchiodi, C. A. (2007). *The art therapy sourcebook* (2nd ed.). McGraw-Hill.
47. Butler, L. D., & McClain-Meeder, K. (2015). Self-care starter kit. Retrieved from http://www.socialwork.buffalo.edu/students/self-care/index.asp

Bartholomew Learns about Diabetes

Belinda J. Dean

Objectives

At the end of this chapter, you will be able to:

- Reflect on the complex emotional needs of a child with a new chronic medical diagnosis.
- Consider best practice health teaching to support the newly diagnosed child and their family through play-based modalities.
- Understand play-based techniques for blood glucose testing and assisting the child along with their family to assist with emotional regulation.

Introduction

One of the primary roles of the nurse or allied health professional is to educate newly diagnosed patients and their families on the complexities of their condition. Many best practice guidelines contribute to informing health teaching across many areas of health care. However, further research is required to create pediatric-specific best practice guidelines for each area of practice. Health teaching should consider the age and stage of development of the pediatric patient being taught. Play-based education is considered developmentally appropriate for children as play is a child's way of understanding their world. Therapeutic play or play-based approaches should be considered as a tailored approach to support the newly diagnosed child and their family to process concerns related to the chronic condition. Thus far, there is little research outlining the benefits of age-appropriate play-based health

B. J. Dean (✉)

School of Health and Social Development, Deakin University, Geelong, VIC, Australia

e-mail: belinda.dean@deakin.edu.au

© The Author(s), under exclusive license to Springer Nature Switzerland AG 2022

J. A. Parson et al. (eds.), *Integrating Therapeutic Play Into Nursing and Allied Health Practice*, https://doi.org/10.1007/978-3-031-16938-0_14

education. The use of age-appropriate play-based techniques support the child and family to build trust in the health care professional and limit the likelihood of iatrogenic (treatment related) trauma in relation to the admission. The following sections outline Batholomew's experience of being newly diagnosed with DM1. Theoretical underpinnings which outline how the diagnosis will impact Bartholomew and his family are then discussed. Finally, how play-based education and therapeutic support will allow Bartholomew and his family to manage his new condition is explored.

Batholomew's Background

Bartholomew is a 10-year-old boy who lives at home with his Mum, Alera, his Mumma, Katrina, and his 11-year-old sister, Zehra. Alera explained that Bartholomew was conceived through in vitro fertilization (IVF) and she carried him through to 38 weeks. Despite spending some time in the special care nursery Katrina described Bartholomew as a well and content baby. Preceding the onset of symptoms, there were no known traumatic experiences for Bartholomew or his family. Alera and Katrina described Bartholomew as a typically developing child who met expected health and developmental milestones. Bartholomew has been diagnosed with type 1 diabetes (DM1) after an episode of diabetic ketoacidosis (DKA). There is no known family history of DM1, however, Katrina and Alera discussed that they do not have an in-depth health history of the sperm donor for Bartholomew. Bartholomew and his family will be provided with health education and psychological support to manage his condition prior to being discharged.

Background to the Clinical Setting through the Eyes of the Child: Batholomew's Experience

Bartholomew reflects on how he ended up lying in this cold, stiff hospital bed.....He thinks maybe he was brought into hospital because he was constantly hungry and thirsty and kept needing to wee and last night, he wet the bed. He thought back and had not done this since he was 3 years old. Bartholomew went red even thinking about it, and felt so embarrassed, he could not believe he passed out too. Bartholomew had been at a sleepover at his best friend Freddie's house when he became very unwell, wet the bed, and became unconscious. Bartholomew remembered that Freddie had said that his breath smelt like lollies even though they'd only had a bag of skittles and some chips. He also remembered he started vomiting everywhere. The next thing Bartholomew knew an ambulance had arrived and there were people all around him, including Freddie, Freddie's parents, and lots of people in uniforms. He remembered falling in and out of sleep and ending up in the kid's ward of the hospital. The ward was so noisy and busy which made his head hurt and his eyes feel even more blurry than they had been for the past few months. Bartholomew felt so tired and just wanted to sleep, however, people kept coming in to take blood from his finger which really hurt. They put a tight squeezy thing on his arm and another thing on his finger that didn't hurt but made him jump every time they went near his finger, and it made so many noises. The worst thing though, Bartholomew reflected, was the needles they kept jabbing into his tummy which hurt the most. They said he had to keep having needles or a pump permanently inserted with a needle. This just made Bartholomew feel sad. He also felt so confused that the nurses and doctors and other staff kept talking about his sugar and he did not have any idea what that meant. He could not believe people really had sugar in their bodies. One person in a white coat said he would never be able to eat lollies again, even at birthday parties. He thought this was a cruel trick and someone would have to pop out soon to tell him he had been pranked. He thought how this was the worst day ever. They even sent his Mumma and Zehra home, only allowing his Mum to stay the night. He felt so scared, believing he would wet the bed again, and did not sleep at all. He was worried that Freddie would hate him or tell everyone at school he was a weirdo baby who wets the bed, vomits, and blacks out for no reason. He was already seen as being different and this was going to make it a billion times worse. He was also worried about all the sport and school he would miss because the doctor had said he cannot go back to school for ages and must stay in hospital until he understands how this thing called diabetes works. He thought there was no way he'd make the basketball team now. He did think that some of the people that had come in to teach him about diabetes had been nice. He especially liked the staff who "got him" and played games with him or drew with him, it made things not as scary.

Activity

Consider Bartholomew's experience. How might he be feeling? How would you feel if you were him? Given he is 10 years old boy, would he still want his family to be with him? What is he experiencing from the environment around him? How overwhelmed is he by the sights, sounds, smells, things touching him, and different food he is tasting? With your current understanding of diabetes, how would his diagnosis be altering his sensations and experience?

Diabetes Mellitus

Diabetes mellitus type 1 (DM1) is known to be one of the fastest growing and most significant chronic health conditions experienced by children [1]. Australian data shows that there is between 500–600 new cases of type 1 diabetes each year in Australian children aged 0–14 years [2]. Currently, over six thousand Australian children experience DM1, which is the sixth highest incidence of new cases world-wide [3]. DM1 is defined as a chronic autoimmune disease in which insulin-producing cells of the pancreas are attacked by the person's immune system, resulting in the cells not being able to produce their own insulin [3]. The Australian Institute of Health and Welfare found that DM1 can occur at any time throughout one's lifespan, however, statistics show that approximately half of all new cases are diagnosed in childhood aged between 0 and 14 years.

Being diagnosed with and living with DM1 in childhood results in ongoing stress and potentially medical trauma which can impact significantly on all areas of bio-logical and psychosocial functioning for the child as well as their family [4]. The Royal Children's Hospital, Melbourne (N.D.) states that obtaining a diagnosis of

T1DM can impact the whole family and brings about much uncertainty and fear for families. Forgey and Bursch [4] describe iatrogenic (treatment related) trauma being triggered through receiving a serious chronic diagnosis such as DM1. Hart and Rollins [5] elaborate on this discussing that both the diagnosis as well as ongoing invasive medical procedures for the remainder of the child's life, can result in ongoing negative psychological and emotional implications. DM1 has been linked to a higher incidence of depression, eating disorders, anxiety, and psychological distress in young people compared to typically developing peers [6]. The ongoing dysregulation of the stress response system results in a toxic stress response which in turn results in negative health outcomes in adulthood [7]. Burke Harris et al. describe this exposure to toxic stress in childhood as an adverse childhood experience (ACE). The more ACEs a child experiences, the greater the risk of having comorbid chronic health conditions into adulthood [8]. Felitti [9] found through the ACEs study that childhood diabetes is a causative factor of later adult physical and psychological illness. DeCosta, Skinner and Grabowski [10] speak of trust at the time of diagnosis as being central to the child's psychosocial experience and the negative impacts of a lack of trusting relationships with healthcare professionals. Play-based approaches at the time of diagnosis and throughout treatment are thought to increase trust and minimize the impacts of traumatic stress for the child and their family [11].

Despite DM1 being a non-modifiable childhood risk factor in relation to ACEs, the management of the condition as well as the modification of stress and strain on the family unit through the establishment of trusting relationships can improve health outcomes. Age-appropriate psychosocial and health education including play-based health teaching, procedural play therapy, medical play therapy, child-centered play therapy, non-directive play therapy, and filial play therapy serve as a protective factor to buffer against the negative impact of ACEs on long-term health outcomes [12]. Burke Harris et al. [7] suggest that to prevent ACEs, research, intervention, and policy are required. Further, Burke Harris et al. suggest that these domains be achieved through the education of families (primary prevention) as well as early detection and intervention (secondary prevention). The authors suggest that appropriate clinical management of childhood diseases results in improved physiological effects from the impacts of early adversity (tertiary prevention). Collaborative care from a multidimensional team is also vital to support the optimal development of the newly diagnosed child [11].

In the field of play therapy, it is widely accepted that play is the language of the child [5, 13, 14] and play-based teaching is the most appropriate means of providing health education and psychosocial support. Despite optimal health teaching and play-based management potentially requiring an increase in time and resources, the capacity-building of patients and their families results in positive outcomes [15]. Patients who are masters of their condition can thrive independently, confidently managing their condition without the need for continual tertiary services. Early intervention through age-appropriate, play-based psychosocial, and health education will result in ensuring that those with a diagnosis of DM1 are able to achieve a long-term healthy integrated sense of self to live optimally with DM1.

Hart and Rollins [5] cite the importance of health teaching at the level of a child's cognitive ability and advises that play is considered of upmost importance to assist children being able to understand the medical experience. Yogman et al. [16]

emphasized the importance of play to reduce stress related to life transitions such as receiving a diagnosis of diabetes. It is hypothesized that if a child is not included in the health teaching for their diagnosis or the health teaching is not pitched at the appropriate age and stage of developmental learning, feelings of isolation, shame, and stress increase the likelihood of behavioral issues and non-compliance with treatment [16, 17]. Creative play acts as a conduit allowing children to express their concerns, problem solve, and process their emotions, it is also an appropriate method for health education [18].

There is little mention in the literature of which strategies are used in health teaching for children and if they are age and stage appropriate such as play-based teaching [19]. Current research reveals that most diabetes education is not standardized [20]. Balderrama [21] provides a clinical checklist for health teaching that is supported by published guidelines providing information on what patient education entails for the child or adolescent with DM1, how this should be administered, where education occurs, and who provides the education [22]. This health teaching and checklist is focused on educational topics such as definitions of DM1, insulin therapy, exercise, diet, and potential complications [21]. It also covers checkpoints such as ensuring privacy, introducing oneself, assessing the patient's readiness to learn, considering barriers to learning and the child's learning desires and priorities, and the individual's preferred learning style. However, the checklist does not mention age-appropriate learning or play-based learning. Likewise, Lange, Swift, Pańkowska, and Danne [23] cite the importance of universal learning principles and state that every child or young person has a right to expert structured comprehensive education. Education should empower the young person to manage their diabetes and should be personalized and age appropriate. Despite outlining the importance of age-appropriate education based on maturity neither the checklist nor the universal language principles mention play-based learning [23]. Lange et al. [23] further cite the importance of the entire family needing to be motivated to learn.

Working from a therapeutic play-based lens, one can consider the underlying play therapy theory that places the child at the center of the experience. Play therapists work from a humanistic stance and use specific techniques and strategies to improve the overall functioning of the child [14, 24]. A humanistic play-based approach is based on Carl Rogers's constructs of personality and the therapy conditions which support growth [13, 25]. Rogers describes the importance of the therapist demonstrating empathy and unconditional positive regard for the child (client) and creating a positive relationship. Axline [26] emphasized the importance of being with the child and revised Roger's foundations to develop non-directive play therapy. The below activity provides an example of a medical model approach to teaching where the health teaching is based solely on the condition compared to one which encompasses humanistic principles and takes a whole systems approach including the family in health teaching as well as Batholomew in a play-based developmentally sensitive way.

Activity—Try to guess which of the below health teaching methods is a traditional teaching method for Bartholomew and which is based on humanistic principles and play. Discuss why you chose the option you did and the pros and cons of each teaching method (Table 1).

Table 1 Health teaching activity

Health teaching activity	Option 1	Option 2
Fingerstick glucose test	Nurse Lisa rushes into the room complaining about how busy her day is and how the boy in room 12 has just taken up all of her time. She comes at a time when Bartholomew is by himself because his family has gone to get a coffee and snacks. Nurse Lisa says, "I know you wanted your family here, but this is the only time I've got and you're 10, you should be fine." She shows Bartholomew the lancet and says "remember this, it's for the finger prick" and then gets his finger and presses it in hard and says "remember I told you last time how you have to press this and then the blood comes out and you put it on the testing strip which is inserted into this machine" She pricks his finger mid-sentence and he gets a sharp sting…. "Oh, and don't forget to calibrate the machine first or it won't work" … "Got it?" She goes on to say, "I already did it this morning so it will be fine, but don't forget next time." Nurse Lisa then says, "now you wait until the machine tells you the reading and then you should know what to do by now about your level, this is the basic stuff, if you don't know this by now, you're in trouble, you've got a whole lifetime of this you know." Nurse Lisa walks quickly away saying "I've got to go but you can ask me any questions you've got when I come back later."	Nurse James waits until the whole family is in the room with Bartholomew as per Bartholomew's wishes to learn with his Mum and sister present so they can help in case he forgets anything. Nurse James speaks to Bartholomew about how his day has been, and how well his football team did this weekend. It turns out they go for the same team, so they have a little cheer together. James also speaks to Alera, Katrina, and Zehra about what they have been up to. James asks Bartholomew if he remembers the special handshake and clap game and song, they made together last time and they do that and laugh. Zehra wants to join in, so they all do it again together. Nurse James then gets Bartholomew to look at all the laid out equipment to see if he remembers what any of it is. He then says they are going to play a memory game and he asks Bartholomew to cover his eyes. He takes one item away and then asks him to open his eyes and tell him what is missing. Bartholomew gets it right every time. He has been practicing and looking forward to this game. Nurse James checks if Bartholomew has any questions before he asks if Bartholomew's ready to perform the magic glove trick (see below) Bartholomew does his magic trick and confidently pricks his finger and puts the drop of blood on the testing strip and waits for his reading.

Case Vignette—*The Child's Experience*

Bartholomew loves it when there are nurses like James, they make the day go quickly and have a good time together. Nurses like Lisa seem scary to Bartholomew, and he feels like he is wasting their time, so he tries to hurry but then he forgets everything and feels anxious and stressed.

Bartholomew is thinking about this as he sees the friendly child life specialist Jess coming over to his hospital bed. He really likes Jess, and he can tell her which staff he likes and those he finds scary. He can also talk to Jess about how his learning is going with all the new stuff he needs to know and mostly how he is feeling. Jess does not always make him talk, sometimes they just play and draw and have fun. Jess told him at the start that what they talk about is private and she does not talk about it to anyone unless it is very serious like Bartholomew feeling extra worried about how someone has treated him or if he is feeling sad and needs help.

Jess told Bartholomew that each time they hung out together they would have some fun activities to do to help him to understand having diabetes. After spending some time chatting together, Jess engaged Bartholomew in several standardized and non-standardized play-based age-appropriate assessments to outline his underlying feelings about his recent diagnosis and hospital stay. Each assessment is detailed below. Following this Jess supported Bartholomew and his family with play-based health teaching to understand his diagnosis as well as techniques to help with the invasive procedure of having to monitor his own blood glucose through using a lancet on his fingertip several times a day. Jess provided support to the professionals involved in Bartholomew's care to ensure play-based teaching was occurring systemically throughout the whole treating team.

Hospital-Based Initial Assessment

Projective assessments can be interpreted with a curious stance to wonder about the meaning of the art or drawing and to contrast and compare it over time with the child to support their representation of themselves at that point in their journey. An example of a projective assessment is a Blob assessment https://www.blobtree.com/ [27]. Blobs are black outlined people-like figure drawings that are printable and allow the child to color which one fits for them. They can assist the child to express their feelings without words. Bartholomew could complete a blob tree to consider how he is feeling about himself and his new diagnosis. He could also complete a blob hospital or blob sick to consider how he is feeling within the hospital environment.

> *First, Jess asked me to colour in a picture of a sort of stick figure in a tree or on the ground. I picked the one of the guy hanging onto the tree branch because I sort of feel like, 'I'm just hanging in there'. I coloured the hands red because I have so many finger pricks and then I left the rest blank because I couldn't pick what colour I was. Then I did one of stick figures in hospital, I picked the one in the bed talking to someone else sitting on the bed, that*

reminded me of how nice Jess is. Then I picked a sick one and I picked the one that had its arms folded and a cloud over its head because I feel really grumpy and have a headache.

An example of a standardized play assessment that the play therapist could engage Bartholomew in is, The Affect in Play Scale (APS) or the brief rating version (APS-BR) of the Affect in Play scale [28, 29]. The Affect in Play scale is a standardized tool with a criterion-based rating scale that measures the child's level of pretend play, divergent thinking, and emotional memories. Through assessing the play of a child, one can understand their functioning or adaptive functioning as well as emotional (affect) expression [18, 30]. The APS is appropriate for children aged 6–10 years old. The APS or APS-BR is appropriate for a hospital setting and could be conducted at the bedside. It contains two human puppets (a girl and a boy) and three brightly coloured different-shaped blocks which are all laid out on a table [29]. The assessment only takes 5 min, making it a suitable tool for a child who is not well. Full instructions on administering the Affect in Play Scale can be found in Russ's book Platy in Child Development and Psychotherapy as an Appendix [30].

The amount and type of affective expressions in Bartholomew's play can be measured as well as themes that may be related to how Bartholomew is experiencing both his new diagnosis and the hospital stay in general [18]. Categories of affect range from happiness to fear and anxiety to disappointment. Affect categories are classified as positive or negative which is helpful to gain an understanding of how Bartholomew is currently coping.

At first, I thought I was a bit big to play with dolls, but it was actually really fun. I had fun with the girl and boy puppet and even got a bit silly which Jess was ok with. I pretended the girl doll tripped over one of the blocks and the boy doll laughed at her and she cried but then he went to help her.

An additional projective assessment is to have Bartholomew draw a picture (spontaneous or impromptu) and ask a range of open inquiry-based questions which provide context around Bartholomew's presentation as well as what may be present within the metaphor of the picture [31]. Drawings could then be continued each week with inquiry-based questions to gain an ongoing understanding of Bartholomew's processing over time. Utilizing drawing as a method for health teaching is an appropriate age-based method for ensuring Bartholomew understands his condition.

Jess said, I could draw a picture of myself, then she asked me all about it. I drew a skinny boy with eyes going round and round in circles stuck in a bed with a sad face and pin pricks all over like sharp rain falling from the roof. She then asked me lots of questions about this and I explained why I might be feeling like that and what it means to have diabetes and how it might impact my body, brain and mood.

Intervention and Health Teaching Support

Russ [32] discusses the link between creativity and flexibility of thinking which impact and are impacted by affect. Being able to engage in creative activities such as drawing, allows Bartholomew to express himself non-verbally giving rise to emotions that may not be on the surface as well as providing a platform for exploring and conveying his worries and concerns to his family and treating team [33]. Drawing can be utilized as projective assessments but can extend to ongoing play-based work with hospital-based children as a tool for communication, as a rapport-building technique, as age-appropriate health teaching and to aid exploration of experiences through inquiry-based questioning [31, 33].

> *Each week we had time together drawing and talking. Jess asked me all about my drawings in ways no one had ever asked me before, it really made me feel like she was interested and actually made some things make sense for me too. She then taught me so much about having diabetes and I really feel like I understand it now. I've got a long way to go but I know who I can ask for help if I need.*

Strategies for Blood Glucose Monitoring

The magic glove is a hypno-anesthetic technique that can limit nociception for a child who is having a painful procedure to their fingers, hands, or arms. The trained health care professional intentionally and repetitively uses physically calculated touch on the patients' fingers, hands, and arms mimicking putting on a glove which is called a magic glove [34]. Suggestive phrases are used to support the outcome of having an altered perception and sensation in the area such as numbness to limit the pain [34]. The technique as well as limiting pain can also minimize anticipatory anxiety which is useful when needing to have ongoing blood glucose monitoring through pricking the finger with a lancet [35].

> *It felt a bit funny when Jess started pretending to put a glove on my hand and said things over and over like, I know what is happening, but I'm not bothered, as I know my glove is protecting my hand. But then when I had to do my next finger prick it didn't even hurt! It was really magic; I actually can't get over it and think I have special magic powers now.*

Systemic Considerations

A systemic approach is vital when considering the impacts of iatrogenic trauma. Levine and Kline [36] discuss medical and surgical procedures as being the most overlooked area when considering the impacts of childhood trauma. When a child is unprepared, is overwhelmed, is restrained, or separated from their caregivers, long-term trauma can be held within the body unless a way to discharge the charge is found. Levine and Kline [36] discuss the latency period of trauma and how it can last from months to years or even decades if not dealt with at the time. Forgey and Bursch [4] cite chronic illness being a risk for frightening experiences within health care settings that can result in iatrogenic trauma. Some situations include receiving a serious diagnosis, managing unfamiliar medical technologies, having painful or distressing procedures, and not having a parent present to support the child. Despite professionals not causing harm intentionally, non-patient-centered models do not allow the child to have a voice or time care at their pace. Parents too can feel powerless in such a system. ISPAD guidelines recommend professionals be patient centered and have specialized training to deliver successful behavioral approaches to parents and children with an interdisciplinary team who speak with one voice to obtain both psychosocial and metabolic outcomes [6, 17]. However, this is not always representative of actual practice. It is important that health care professionals take on a systems approach and allow the voice of the child to be heard to ensure best practices.

Levine and Kline [36] discuss strategies to avoid trauma as well as first aid for exposure to iatrogenic trauma. Parents can be proactive by firstly aiming to find a treating team who are trauma informed. Secondly, parents can remain calm and regulate themselves. If parents and children both know what to expect they will be able to stay more regulated. Parents who are informed can be even more helpful and less anxious regarding medical procedures such as diabetic monitoring [22]. Levine and Kline [36] discuss that children should never be strapped down or anesthetized when in a terrified state and should not wake up from esthetic alone as both could cause imprinting of trauma due to an undischarged freeze response that increases the risk of traumatic stress and PTSD. Parents will feel more able to advocate for their child if they feel empowered from the beginning.

Recognizing potential trauma symptoms such as the child being hyper-vigilant, clingy, fearful, withdrawn, angry, or impulsive or experiencing incontinence, headaches, nightmares, or stomach pains is important to allow the parent to find ways to ameliorate the traumatic response. DeCosta, Grabowski, and Skinner [10] report on depressive symptoms being linked to a reaction to being newly diagnosed. Some examples include depressed mood, irritability, social withdrawal, and feeling anxious. They also report on PTSD symptoms at the time of diagnosis and discuss that 4.3%–5.4% of the children studied displayed moderate to severe post-traumatic stress symptoms. Levine and Kline [36] report that post-traumatic reactions may remain dormant unless it is dealt with. Levine and Kline [36] provide a step-by-step parent guide to manage a traumatic response, the first steps are listed below as examples. See resource below for full details.

1. Check-in with your own body first (to be sure you are regulated).
2. Assess what traumatic symptoms the child has and allow time to rest.
3. Guide the child to experience and speak about their bodily sensations (How do you feel in your tummy? What color, shape, and size is that feeling?).
4. Be slow and follow the pace of the child, allow the child time to process and release their big feelings. Know when they may have processed the big feelings and are out of the traumatic state. They may start to smile, yawn, stretch, or breathe more slowly.
5. Allow the child to have whatever reaction they need to have. Avoid saying "*it's all going to be ok*" and allow them to cry and tremble to discharge the freeze response and reassure them those feelings are good to come out.

Chapter Summary

Intragenic trauma may occur at the time of diagnosis for a newly diagnosed child. However, using age-appropriate play-based techniques assist the child and family to build trust with professionals which may improve health outcomes. It also allows for experiences to be processed and integrated resulting in a reduction in the likelihood of experiencing traumatic stress. As the professional working with a newly diagnosed child and family, considering best practice health teaching with a play-based approach is crucial as is ensuring play-based techniques are used to facilitate invasive procedures such as blood glucose testing. A multidisciplinary approach that includes the family and child as part of the system will ensure best practice in care, health teaching, and minimizing the impacts of iatrogenic trauma due to a new diagnosis.

Additional Resources

The Magic Glove—Hypnotic plain management for children—https://www.youtube.com/watch?v=cyApK8Z_SQQ
   PDF of the Magic Glove from Dr. Leora Kuttner:

https://pediatric-pain.ca/wp-content/uploads/2013/04/The_Magic_Glove12.pdf

   First aid for trauma:

Peter A. Levine, Ph.D, Maggie Kline (2007) Trauma Through a Child's Eyes: Awakening the Ordinary Miracle of Healing.
Peter Levine website: https://www.somaticexperiencing.com/se-interviews

References

1. Kise, S. S., Hopkins, A., & Burke, S. (2017). Improving school experiences for adolescents with type 1 diabetes. *The Journal of School Health, 87*(5), 363–375. https://doi.org/10.1111/josh.12507
2. Australian Institute of Health and Welfare. (2020). Data tables: Incidence of insulin-treated diabetes in Australia 2020. In A. I. o. H. a. Welfare (Ed.). Australian Institute of Health and Welfare.
3. Australian Institute of Health and Welfare. (2015). Prevalence of type 1 diabetes among children aged 0–14 in Australia 2013. 2019, from https://www.aihw.gov.au/reports/diabetes/type1-diabetes-among-children-aged-0-14-2013/contents/table-of-contents
4. Forgey, M., & Bursch, B. (2013). Assessment and management of pediatric iatrogenic medical trauma. *Current Psychiatry Reports*, 15(2), 340. https://doi.org/10.1007/s11920-012-0340-5
5. Hart, R., & Rollins, J. (2011). *Therapeutic activities for children and teens coping with health issues*. John Wiley & Sons.
6. Delamater, A. M., de Wit, M., McDarby, V., Malik, J. A., Hilliard, M. E., Northam, E., & Acerini, C. L. (2018). ISPAD Clinical Practice Consensus Guidelines 2018: Psychological care of children and adolescents with type 1 diabetes. *Pediatric Diabetes, S27*, 237. https://doi.org/10.1111/pedi.12736

7. Burke Harris, N., Silvério Marques, S., Oh, D., Bucci, M., & Cloutier, M. (2017). Prevent, screen, heal: Collective action to fight the toxic effects of early life adversity. *Academic Pediatrics, 17*(7), S14–S15. https://doi.org/10.1016/j.acap.2016.11.015

8. Dube, S. R., Fairweather, D., Pearson, W. S., Felitti, V. J., Anda, R. F., & Croft, J. B. (2009). Cumulative childhood stress and autoimmune diseases in adults. *Psychosomatic Medicine, 71*(2), 243–250. https://doi.org/10.1097/PSY.0b013e3181907888

9. Felitti, V. J. (2002). The relation between adverse childhood experiences and adult health: Turning gold into lead. *The Permanente Journal, 6*(1), 44–47.

10. DeCosta, P., Grabowski, D., & Skinner, T. C. (2020). The psychosocial experience and needs of children newly diagnosed with type 1 diabetes from their own perspective: a systematic and narrative review. *Diabetic Medicine, 37*(10), 1640. https://doi.org/10.1111/dme.14354.

11. Marshall, L., & DeMarie, D. (2021). Integration of play therapy in medical settings: Understanding the link between mental health and medical health. *International Journal of Play Therapy, 30*(3), 167–176. https://doi.org/10.1037/pla0000165

12. Larkin, H., Shields, J. J., & Anda, R. F. (2012). The health and social consequences of adverse childhood experiences (ACE) across the lifespan: An introduction to prevention and intervention in the community. *Journal of Prevention & Intervention in the Community, 40*(4), 263–270. https://doi.org/10.1080/10852352.2012.707439

13. Schaefer, C. E. (2011). *Foundations of play therapy*. Wiley. ©2011. 2nd ed.

14. Schaefer, C. E., & Drewes, A. A. (2014). *The therapeutic powers of play: 20 core agents of change* (2nd ed.). John Wiley & Sons, Inc.

15. Goodridge, D., McDonald, M., New, L., Scharf, M., Harrison, E., Rotter, T., et al. (2019). Building patient capacity to participate in care during hospitalisation: A scoping review. *BMJ Open, 9*, 7. https://doi.org/10.1136/bmjopen-2018-026551

16. Yogman, M., Garner, A., Hutchinson, J., Hirsh-Pasek, K., Golinkoff, R. M., Baum, R., et al. (2018). The power of play: A pediatric role in enhancing development in young children. *Pediatrics, 142*, 3. https://doi.org/10.1542/peds.2018-2058

17. Phelan, H., Lange, K., Cengiz, E., Gallego, P., Majaliwa, E., Pelicand, J., et al. (2018). ISPAD Clinical Practice Consensus Guidelines 2018: Diabetes education in children and adolescents. *Pediatric Diabetes, S27*, 75. https://doi.org/10.1111/pedi.12762

18. Russ, S. W. (2004b). *Play in child development and psychotherapy: Toward empirically supported practice*. Lawrence Erlbaum.

19. The Royal Children's Hospital Melbourne (n.d.). Clinical Practice Guidelines Diabetes mellitus. Retrieved 19th June 2019, from https://www.rch.org.au/clinicalguide/guideline_index/Diabetes_Mellitus/.

20. Ramchandani, N., Johnson, K., Cullen, K., Hamm, T., Bisordi, J., & Sullivan-Bolyai, S. (2017). CDE perspectives of providing New-onset type 1 diabetes education using formal vignettes and simulation. *The Diabetes Educator, 43*(1), 97–104. https://doi.org/10.1177/0145721716676893

21. Balderrama, D. R. M. (2017). *Patient education: Teaching the child or adolescent with diabetes mellitus, type 1 -- interactive*. EBSCO Publishing.

22. Schub, T. B., & Smith, N. R. M. C. (2017). *Patient education: Teaching the child or adolescent with diabetes mellitus, type 1*. EBSCO Publishing.

23. Lange, K., Swift, P., Pańkowska, E., & Danne, T. (2014). ISPAD Clinical Practice Consensus Guidelines 2014. Diabetes education in children and adolescents. *Pediatric Diabetes, 15*(Suppl 20), 77–85. https://doi.org/10.1111/pedi.12187

24. Drewes, A. A., & Schaefer, C. E. (2014). How play therapy causes therapeutic change. In C. E. Schaefer & A. A. Drewes (Eds.), *The therapeutic powers of play: 20 core agents of change* (2nd ed.). John Wiley & Sons, Inc.

25. Rogers, C. R. (2007). The necessary and sufficient conditions of therapeutic personality change. *Psychotherapy: Theory, Research, Practice, Training, 44*(3), 240–248.

26. Axline, V. M. (1969). *Play therapy*. Ballantine Books.

27. Wilson, P., & Long, I. (2018). The big book of blob trees. Updated (2nd ed.). New York: Routledge. Updated.

28. Cordiano, T. J. S., Russ, S. W., & Short, E. J. (2008). Development and validation of the affect in play scale-brief rating version (APS-BR). *Journal of Personality Assessment, 90*(1), 52–60. https://doi.org/10.1080/00223890701693744

29. Russ, S. W. (2014). *Pretend play in childhood: Foundation of adult creativity.* American Psychological Association.

30. Russ, S. W. (2004a). Appendix: Affect in play scale. In S. W. Russ (Ed.), *Play in child development and psychotherapy: Toward empirically supported practice* (pp. 145–155). Lawrence Erlbaum.

31. Yasenik, L. (2021). *Inquiry skills with children and youth.*

32. Russ, S. W. (2013). *Affect and creativity: The role of affect and play in the creative process.* Taylor and Francis.

33. Malchiodi, C. A., & Goldring, E. (2013). Art therapy and child life. In C. A. Malchiodi (Ed.), *Art therapy and health care.* Guilford Press.

34. Coogle, J., Coogle, B., & Quezada, J. (2021). Hypnosis in the treatment of pediatric functional neurological disorder: The magic glove technique. *Pediatric Neurology, 125*, 20–25. https://doi.org/10.1016/j.pediatrneurol.2021.08.011

35. Kuttner, L. (2012). Pediatric hypnosis: Pre-, peri-, and post-anesthesia. *Pediatric Anesthesia, 22*(6), 573–577. https://doi.org/10.1111/j.1460-9592.2012.03860.x

36. Levine, P., & Kline, M. (2007). *Trauma through a child's eyes: Awakening the ordinary miracle of healing.* North Atlantic Books.

Charlotte's Hospice Stay: Time for Play

Erin Butler

Objectives

At the end of this chapter, you will be able to:

- Reflect on the complex emotional needs of a child with a life-limiting illness and their family.
- Develop a basic understanding of holistic play development, core conditions of play and principles of CCPT.
- Review strategies for supporting a terminally ill or dying child and their family through play, using knowledge of holistic play development, core conditions and CCPT principles to inform practice.
- Self-reflect on the important role the reader holds within their practice and the future relationships they form with this demographic and their families.
- Consider self-care strategies to support emotional wellness when providing end-of-life care.

When reality is painful and a child's future not bright, we may sometimes be tempted to feel that it is kinder to leave a child in a state of not being able to think… This would be to deny the very humanity of the child and their right to a full life, whatever it may hold and however brief it may be.—McMahon [1]:165

E. Butler (✉)
Sydney, NSW, Australia
e-mail: playtherapywitherin@gmail.com

J. A. Parson et al. (eds.), *Integrating Therapeutic Play Into Nursing and Allied Health Practice*, https://doi.org/10.1007/978-3-031-16938-0_15

Introduction

A life-limiting illness can be defined as a condition or disease which has no reasonable expectation of a cure and is fatal [2]. The premature death of a child can be caused by a range of different diagnoses, some of which are related to congenital abnormalities, muscular disorders, organ failure, metabolic conditions, severe multiple disabilities or neurodegenerative and neurological conditions [3]. An illness may oscillate between being perceived as chronic or life-limiting, depending on numerous factors which determine the clinical course of the condition and the prognosis. Such factors can vary greatly depending on the cause, stability, predictability and complexity of the illness. These characteristics can determine whether the life-limiting illness is degenerative or immediately threatening and how demanding or restricting it can be for the child [4].

With technology and modern medicine continually evolving, children who might have died from a particular illness decades ago are now more likely to live healthier, productive lives [5]. However, depending on the diagnosis and prognosis of the child's illness, they could be faced with significant healthcare treatment over varying periods of time and sadly, eventually their own death. With the medical profession actively working towards the prevention and cure of childhood illness, a reduction of the physical, social, and psychological impacts is also a high priority [6]. When children have been diagnosed with a life-limiting illness, a holistic approach to their health care is necessary to ensure that both their pain is controlled and symptoms are managed, but also their emotional well-being is addressed [7].

The diagnosis of a life-limiting illness can result in the child and their family experiencing a range of stressors, particularly in relation to how their illness is managed [5]. Locating adequate health care and support services for long-term management may contribute to the stress experienced, along with factors such as financial burden, uncertainty of the future, and a subsequent increase in family tension. Living with a life-limiting illness can result in the child not being able to utilise their natural coping behaviours, due to experiencing high levels of stress, pain and anxiety [8]. As each experience of physical illness will vary, the provision of appropriate support should be unique to the needs of the child and all involved with supporting the child to enhance the likelihood of coping, understanding and adjustment.

Upon diagnosis, most children with a life-limiting illness will be admitted to hospital and then will intermittently return for medical treatment throughout their lifetime, depending on the illness, condition or disease [9]. Some may even attend a children's hospice for occasional respite or end-of-life care. Anxiety, tension, medical procedures, financial strain, uncertainty, and reliance on support services or other personnel are just some of the experiences that may have a negative individual or collective impact [5].

With a limited number of children's hospices Australia-wide and many children geographically dispersed, there is a need for paediatric palliative care services to improve the quality of life for children experiencing life-limiting conditions and their families by providing specialised support in the home or hospital [10, 11]. This chapter will draw on the author's own research, professional experience and relevant literature to determine how therapeutic play or CCPT can be effective, holistic, safe and supportive for children living with a life-limiting illness. It will also explore how the therapeutic relationship is of importance when supporting the child and the family unit. Whilst this chapter will be focusing on the therapist's role in the context of a children's hospice, the reader is encouraged to reflect on the role that they hold within their current practice and how they can apply this knowledge to further enhance the relationships and quality of life of the children and families that they encounter.

A Progressive Brain Tumour—Charlotte's Experience

Charlotte, a 7-year-old Australian girl, with a progressive brain tumour, woke as her family pulled up in the driveway of a place she had not visited before. Charlotte's parents and brothers did not talk very much during the drive so she knew they were worried and sad. Charlotte noticed that she was also feeling nervous because she was not sure what to expect. She had heard about this place called a children's hospice and wondered whether it would be like her experience of being in the hospital. In the hospital, there were lots of people constantly coming and going from her shared room, her surroundings were not familiar, and her family could not be together all the time. Charlotte felt her heart race and a heavy feeling in her stomach, she really hoped she would like it here because she knew things were getting very tough for her body. The simplest things she used to find easy to do, such as breathing, talking, remembering things and walking, were becoming increasingly more challenging as her condition deteriorated further. A friendly nurse came to greet Charlotte and her family in the car park and Charlotte was transferred to her wheelchair. She took some deep breaths as she was wheeled through the doors and into the lift with her family. Her Mum reassuringly rubbed her arm, and the lift made a 'ding' sound. The first thing Charlotte saw as the doors opened were lots of children's photos and artworks on the walls—it already seemed like a special place where so many children had already been, and this comforted Charlotte a little.

As they entered the corridor, they were welcomed with a play space, which looked like there were lots of options of things to play with and do. The nurse introduced Charlotte to the Child Life Therapist/ Play Therapist, Lexi, then continued to show her where her room was going to be. Charlotte could not believe it! A whole room all to herself with an adjoining room where her family could also sleep. She noticed on her door there was a specially crafted name sign, on her bed there was a cosy quilt, and, on the shelves, there seemed to be lots of things that she really enjoyed, like art materials, books to read and a variety of games. Charlotte looked out the window and beyond the sunny balcony she saw some beautiful trees, a garden and the sea in the distance. The pit in her stomach seemed to have eased and this place began to feel a little more like home… In the days and weeks that followed, Charlotte's parents and brothers did not leave her side. They spoke of all kinds of things—recalled memories, shared photos, videos and laughed together. They also made plans of what things they could do during their stay, such as visit the beach, eat ice cream, make family artworks, spend time in the garden, listen to music and play together as a family. Charlotte knew she was dying and tried so very hard to be brave and strong for her family, but sometimes she just felt like crying. Inside, Charlotte felt really scared because she was so sick, in pain and completely exhausted. She desperately wished things were different. Something that helped with these big feelings, was spending time with Lexi. Lexi always came up with fun ideas of what Charlotte and her brothers could do, which also gave her Mum and Dad a much-needed break. The more time Charlotte spent with Lexi, the more Charlotte felt safe and knew she could genuinely show all the different sides to herself. This meant, as things became physically more challenging for Charlotte when her condition deteriorated further, there was not an expectation 'to do' lots of things or feel certain ways, but Lexi could 'just be' with her when needed—something that helped Charlotte feel deeply cared for, comforted, understood and accepted, particularly when words became too difficult to form.

Child-Centred Play Therapy

The Child-Centred Play Therapy (CCPT) approach has proven to be an effective intervention for children of different developmental stages, client groups and cultural backgrounds [12]. It has long been known that the theoretical understanding behind CCPT is to enable the child to use their innate ability to strive towards growth, maturity and acceptance through self-directional play [12–14]. With consistent and repeated exposure to sensitive attunement and core therapeutic conditions such as empathy, congruence and unconditional positive regard, a mutually respectful, accepting, permissive and safe relationship evolves between the therapist and child over time [12, 15]. These facilitating elements of the relationship are the main causation for change and growth to occur within the child throughout the therapeutic experience, enabling an experiential, intuitive learning and acceptance of the self to evolve [14].

Whilst living with a life-limiting illness, the child will have a range of emotional needs related to the loss of a fully functioning or physically healthy body, their identity or the experience of vulnerability and dependence on others. Where these children often experience fewer opportunities for self-directed play and control over their lived experiences, CCPT offers them a space to freely lead, set the pace of their sessions and develop mastery [1]. With repeated opportunities for self-awareness and self-developed skills, this supports the process of self-actualisation to occur as it enables the child to completely trust themselves and their feelings, which leads to an overall feeling of peace within [16]. With an understanding of the core conditions and main beliefs that underpin the process of CCPT, the reader can reflect on how they build relationships, engage with children in their care, support children through play experiences and improve outcomes for the children and families they work with.

It is thought that to provide an appropriate and effective therapeutic experience, the therapist should carefully consider the unique needs of each child, regardless of their reasons for referral [5]. Depending on the child's communicative or physical abilities, such as whether they are non-verbal, experience physical limitations or are immobile, therapist expectations and certain adaptations to the therapeutic space and sessions may be necessary [8]. Considering how the space is set up and organised is important to ensure everything is accessible, appropriate and practical for the child, such as ensuring all play items are clearly visible, providing options where play experiences can be brought to the child, and flexible seating or enough room for those in wheelchairs to move freely or fit under tables with ease. The therapist should also be mindful of confidentiality and sensitive to the porous nature of hospital rooms, open play spaces or various areas within the hospice. The lack of privacy may cause the child to feel inhibited, vulnerable or exposed within their therapeutic play process and may also have an impact on the relationship [14]. Acknowledging the space limitations to the child can help create a feeling of containment within the therapeutic relationship.

Another structural consideration for the therapist is to be flexible to the child's needs with each encounter, as some children may require a shorter time with the therapist or may not be able to attend a session at all. This could be due to the ill child being physically unable to sustain a longer session if experiencing physical or mental exhaustion, feeling unwell or experiencing discomfort and pain. However, once children are engaged in play, they are often in a state of flow, where the positive feelings aroused can balance the negative feelings associated with the discomfort or pain they are experiencing [17]. With a holistic understanding of play developmental stages and considering the child's needs and capabilities, the therapist may find that they need to be more directive in some circumstances, such as presenting suitable options to the child using visuals that represent various attachment, somatic sensory, rhythmic, embodiment, projection and role play options for the child to select [18, 19]. Through aiming to acknowledge and attend to the minutest indication of interest and communication such as eye movements, symbols, signing or mirroring, the therapist is also able to establish a connection and maintain the therapeutic relationship [1].

The therapist's choice of materials also needs to be considered and adaptable to the environment that the child is in, particularly if they are in isolation, confined to a bed or require sessions in an alternate setting, such as within the hospital, hospice or home. The provision of carefully chosen toys and materials that are of a sensory, nurturing, real-world, aggressive and creative nature are encouraged as these can further support the child's emotional release, expression, thought processes, and behaviours related to their imminent death [14]. Providing unstructured play materials can also further assist with alleviating the child's anxiety and provides opportunities for regressive play, which can help to soothe and relax the child [1]. A thorough understanding of various types of play, sensory regulation and the developmental needs or interests of the child can further support the child during their stay or in moments of distress, difficulty or pain. Some strategies for consideration could include:

- Breathing, i.e. blowing bubbles, a pin wheel or using 'big belly' breathing with the support of a toy, expanding sphere or shape breathing.

- Physical touch, i.e. comfort positioning, paediatric massage, attachment-based play experiences, sand play, tactile toys or engaging with a therapy pet.
- Sight, i.e. toys that light up, visuals, pictures, bubbles and puppets.
- Sound, i.e. singing familiar songs or musical instrument play, reading children's literature or guided visualisations, tracking and reflecting.
- Smell, i.e. diffusers, mists, essential oils or bringing nature indoors with leaves and flowers.
- Taste, i.e. cooking experiences, eating familiar or comforting food, or drinking cold water (if child can eat or drink orally).

There may also be various spaces, activities and experiences that will enable the therapeutic relationship to be transferred to different contexts, such as a multi-sensory room, lounge room, garden, or a nearby park. Following a child's lead with their interests or wishes within or beyond the hospice grounds can facilitate normalisation, enhance the quality life of the child and help create lasting memories for the family as a whole.

Case Vignette—Charlotte's Experience

When a child, such as Charlotte, lives with a life-limiting illness, they may be affected in a range of ways and varying degrees of severity due to the impact that the illness has on their general health, appearance, mobility, lifestyle and social interactions [20]. Often an ill child can experience a loss of self-control, powerlessness or inadequacy as they are forced to manage daily treatments or numerous medical procedures. This may consequently cause depression, anger, resentment, anxiety or behavioural problems to emerge and can impede aspects of their development or their level of independence [6]. Physiological or emotional regression may also be a challenge, particularly for toddlers or during adolescence, as the loss of newly acquired or firmly established developmental skills need to be re-learned or re-experienced [21].

Niethammer [21] suggests that the illness and the proposed treatment plan should be explored openly with the child in a developmentally appropriate manner. Such consideration to their present understanding, ensures active involvement in the decision-making process occurs. Attempts to protect children from their illness or pending death is thought to be ineffective and potentially harmful, as an ill child is able to respond to their own internal and external cues [22, 23]. CCPT provides a platform for the child to openly explore their treatment plan, condition and potential outcomes in a developmentally appropriate way. Research has been conducted on the various phases that a child will experience during the course of their illness. Depending on their experience, it is believed that each child will process a range of information, issues and tasks during the pre-diagnosis, acute, chronic and terminal phases of their illness [23]. The ways in which a child manages or expresses their wishes, emotions and thoughts surrounding their life-limiting illness can have an overall effect on their self-concept and can be less or more challenging depending on the child's age, what is communicated to them, their level of cognitive understanding and the longevity of the illness before it leads to death [21]. As death is an abstract concept, each child will make sense of their own mortality differently depending on their age or stage of development, revisiting or reforming their understandings throughout their life if the illness is prolonged. To support children with making sense of this complex understanding, they should be provided with opportunities to connect through play as this can naturally offer non-verbal and verbal ways to explore and enhance their understanding of their past or present circumstances and the uncertainty of their future [16].

When children are placed within a hospital environment for medical treatment of their illness, repeated stays may be necessary and could last a matter of days, weeks, months or even years. Hubbuck [24] identified that some of the biggest anxieties experienced during these stays are usually concerned with the treatment method being painful, frightening or unpleasant. These anxieties, combined with the lack of freedom, self-control and privacy, can be experienced at different intensities, depending on the child's cognitive development and the amount of separation from familiar surroundings [5]. Practical improvements to children's wards or hospitals have aided the accommodation of children's needs, such as admission and treatment preparation, flexible visitation hours, the inclusion of play programs? and access to social experiences [9]. Whilst these are valid methods to alleviate anxiety and create a less threatening hospital experience for children, multiple experiences of high stress and painful procedures can cause the ill child to develop mistrust towards medical professionals over time. This is also why the establishment of a safe therapeutic environment and relationship becomes crucial for a child with a life-limiting illness, providing them with a sense of acceptance, freedom of choice, stability and opportunity for mastery [5]. Creating a home-like experience for children and their family within a children's hospice can further support the child and family to experience medical treatment and health care support in a less clinical manner.

It has been found that some children who remain hospitalised for a longer duration may not be well enough to engage in CCPT [25]. There are also some factors that may influence the outcomes of the play-based process such as, prior hospital experience, the child's coping style, timing, parental influence and the developmental stage of the child [26]. Depending on the needs of the child, access to different therapeutic approaches may need to be considered as there may be certain therapies that are more suitable or appropriate. For example, providing Music and Art Therapy within the hospital or hospice setting to children that are physically restricted, severely ill or at the end of their life [27, 28].

The Family Experience

When a child, such as Charlotte, is diagnosed with a life-limiting illness, the entire family unit can be either directly or indirectly affected depending on how the illness is responded to and how much friction or strain is experienced as a result. Changes in parenting, parent–child relationships and hierarchy of family members, may have repercussions on the children in the family, particularly regarding self-concept, personality, emotional responses or social isolation [4]. If the illness is of life-limiting nature, the heightened experience of unrelenting stress, anxiety and anticipatory grief may impede on the parents ability to cope adequately [20]. Other factors that may also impact the family are the ill child's age, developmental understanding, level of comfortability or pain experienced, the location of the setting and whether there is access to a supportive network [20]. A study exploring the concepts of children with chronic illness conducted by Brewster [29], concluded that the coping style of the family can generally be a predictor of how well the child deals with or manages their illness. It has also been found that familial characteristics such as the ability to problem solve, be expressive, low incidence of conflict and satisfaction of medical care, can all contribute to a greater acceptance of and adaptation to the illness [30].

Understandably, when the ill child becomes the priority in the family due to the high demands of their physical health and emotional wellbeing needs, often the siblings will become unacknowledged and unsupported [31]. This can cause possible resentment, anxiety, guilt, jealousy, anger, loneliness or embarrassment to be experienced [32]. Continual experiences of such feelings can lead to the occurrence of socialisation, maladjustment and underachievement issues [33]. Therefore, opportunities for CCPT or therapeutic play can be helpful for the sibling to process and make sense of their own experiences, emotions and grief. With all these complex systemic factors in mind, a therapist's relationship with the family can play an integral role within the therapeutic process [5]. The therapist can actively support the caregivers to improve their overall understanding of their ill child's and other children's emotions, behaviours and adjustment difficulties, whilst providing insight into how they can best support them all throughout the process.

Systemic Approach to Support the Child and Family

Depending on the needs of the family, relevant and suitable support groups or services may also be offered and accessed additionally to CPPT or therapeutic play. A family-centred approach should be priority and can be achieved through thoughtful consideration of how to meet each member's needs. As there is usually a team of health, social and educational professionals involved with each case, a comprehensive and collaborative multidisciplinary approach is necessary to ensure the lives of the ill child and their family are enhanced. Hospitals or hospices may offer psychological or counselling support, Child Life Therapists, Art Therapists, Music Therapists, family support workers, social workers or community support networks to help the entire family manage the various psychological or practical needs and issues [20]. One way the therapist may work towards achieving a holistic, family-centred approach in their clinical practice is through the provision of Filial Therapy sessions. Filial Therapy can support and enhance parent–child relationships within the family using therapeutic principles such as reflection, acceptance and limit setting [34]. A study conducted by Tew [30], reported that parental attitudes towards the illness improved and acceptance of the child increased, whilst a decrease in stress was experienced. Results also demonstrated that children within the family also experienced a lower incidence of behaviour problems, anxiety and depression.

Therapeutic play opportunities centred around memory or legacy making, can also be an inclusive experience for the whole family, supporting each member to play, connect, express their emotions and make lasting memories together. Such experiences can be facilitated by the therapist in collaboration with the family and can consist of various creative expressions or play. Examples include painting art works as a family, creatively incorporating finger, hand or footprints into art works, collecting items or mementos to include in a family memory box or scrap book, taking or collecting photographs to make a collage, jewellery making, crafting family hand moulds, creating a family story or song, documenting family memories into a journal or simply playing games together. Such playful and connected experiences can be considered stress inoculation for the family, supporting them to process their emotions in relation to the ongoing medical treatment and expected loss [17].

Chapter Summary

Play is viewed as a natural way for a child to gain control of their environment and cope with the stressors that are endured when living with a life-limiting illness [25]. Whether the child is in hospital or a hospice, therapeutic play or CCPT should be considered as integral, developmentally appropriate supports. Playful and creative experiences provide the ill or dying child with coping strategies and opportunities to express their complex emotions in a constructive, symbolic and contained way. Through such a holistic and safe process, along with the establishment of a trusting relationship, the child is also able to use play to express, explore and make meaning of their life experience, internal conflicts, thoughts, questions and misunderstandings in relation to their illness, the loss of a healthy body and pending death [14]. Change can occur in several ways as the child begins to integrate their illness into their life, enabling them to experience acceptance, awareness, control, empowerment and mastery [14, 17].

The therapeutic relationship may need to be transferred between various spaces depending on the needs of the ill child, their diagnosis, or prognosis and when medical interventions are necessary. When working with children who have a life-limiting illness, the therapeutic space can be impacted in various ways and certain factors may need to be considered such as time, maintenance of boundaries, privacy and physical alterations or adjustments. At the heart of an effective therapeutic intervention is the therapeutic relationship. Establishing a strong relationship with the child and family can support the 'therapeutic space' to be transferred to any setting or physical space when needed.

The involvement and support of the entire family is crucial throughout the process, from the initial referral/assessment phase through to the eventual ending and beyond. Adopting a family-centred approach with a holistic consideration of each family member's needs is necessary, to ensure the ill child is not being supported in isolation. Establishing strong parental relationships is considered critical, particularly as often there is great complexity within the history, background and relationship dynamics of the family. The therapist plays an integral role in supporting the parents or caregivers to see past the physiological issues that the ill or dying child faces and enables them to comprehend the emotional needs that are present. The disentangling of such difficulties within the family enables the caregiver to consider the perspective of the child's experience. Depending on the family's circumstances and needs, additional support services may need to be accessed in conjunction with therapeutic play or CCPT, to ensure a holistic approach is implemented. The therapist may employ additional skillsets such as Filial Therapy when supporting the family, depending on their needs. Provision of such support can assist with the reparation of various relationships and positively alter the dynamics within the family unit. Other psychological or emotional supports may also be offered or provided to support the caregivers and siblings throughout the intervention.

When working with this demographic, the therapist will need to work as part of a multi-disciplinarian team to achieve a holistic approach with the family involved. In doing so, the therapist can be an advocate for the child and family whilst gaining practical skills and knowledge from other professions. Providing an array of creative interventions such as Music Therapy or Art Therapy, in addition to therapeutic play or CCPT, is important and necessary within a children's hospital as each modality can bring different opportunities to the child and family, particularly towards the end of their life. Consideration of the child's unique needs is necessary when determining which therapeutic support would be most suitable. Finally, whilst it is a privilege and can be deeply rewarding work, when reflecting on one's professional role it is important to consider the practice of regular self-care. This may look different for each person, but it is necessary when engaging in such complex and emotional work. The reader is encouraged to consider what is necessary for nourishing their own wellbeing, whether it be attending to your basic needs of adequate sleep, good nutrition, regular exercise or engaging in social interactions, playful or creative experiences, connecting with nature or attending clinical supervision and personal therapy.

Reflective Questions and Activities

- Reflect on your personal experience of death, grief and loss. How could you use this understanding when interacting with and supporting the emotional needs of the children and families in your care? What might be some triggers for you to be aware of when engaging in this type of work?
- With your understanding of the core conditions of play and principles of Child Centred Play Therapy (CPPT), how do you currently convey your personal qualities and provide a safe space for the children in your care? What could you be more mindful of in your practice?
- Consider how you would support a dying child and their family through play. How could you playfully incorporate connection to the senses to ensure the play

is developmentally appropriate for the child, i.e. sight, sound, smell, taste or touch?

- Reflect on your own self-care practices. What do you currently do to ensure you are supporting and nurturing yourself? What experiences would you like to include in your regular self-care practice?

References

1. McMahon, L. (2009). *The handbook of play therapy and therapeutic play* (2nd ed.). Routledge.
2. Fraser, L. K., Miller, M., Aldridge, J., McKinney, P. A., & Parslow, R. C. (2011). *Life limiting and life threatening conditions in children and young people in the United Kingdom; National and regional prevalence in relation to socioeconomic status and ethnicity. Final report for together for short lives.* Leeds University, Division of Epidemiology. http://www.together-forshortlives.org.uk/assets/0000/1100/Leeds_University___Childr en_s_Hospices_UK_-_Ethnicity_Report.pdf
3. Crowe, L. (2003). *When children have a life limiting illness: Questions and answers around grief and loss.* Centre for Palliative Care Research and Education. https://www.health.qld.gov.au/cpcre/pdf/chldrn_lifelim.pdf
4. Eiser, C. (1993). *Growing up with a chronic disease: The impact on children and their families.* Jessica Kingsley Publishers.
5. Murphy Jones, E. (2001). Play therapy for children with chronic illness. In G. L. Landreth (Ed.), *Innovations in play therapy: Issues, process, and special populations* (pp. 271–288). Routledge.
6. Murphy Jones, E., & Carnes-Holt, K. (2010). The efficacy of intensive individual child centred play therapy for chronically ill children. In J. N. Baggerly, D. C. Ray, & S. C. Bratton (Eds.), *Child-centred play therapy research* (pp. 51–68). John Wiley & Sons.
7. Breeman, C. V. (2009). Using play therapy in paediatric palliative care: Listening to the story and caring for the body. *International Journal of Palliative Nursing, 15*(10), 510–514.
8. Landreth, G. L., Homeyer, L. E., Glover, G., & Sweeney, D. S. (1996). *Play therapy interventions with children's problems.* Jason Aronson Inc.
9. Eiser, C. (1990). *Chronic childhood disease: An introduction to psychological theory and research.* Cambridge University Press.
10. Mherekumombe, M. F., Frost, J., Hanson, S., Shepherd, E., & Collins, J. (2016). Pop up: A new model of paediatric palliative care. *Journal of Paediatrics and Child Health, 52,* 979–982.
11. QuoCCA. (n.d.). *Paediatric palliative care services in Australia.* https://www.quocca.com.au/tabid/4682/Default.aspx
12. Cochran, N. H., Nordling, W. J., & Cochran, J. L. (2010). *Child-centred pay therapy.* John Wiley & Sons.
13. Axline, V. M. (1989). *Play therapy.* Churchill Livingstone.
14. Landreth, G. L. (2012). *Play therapy: The art of the relationship* (3rd ed.). Routledge.
15. Rogers, C. R. (1951). *Client-centred therapy.* Constable & Company Ltd.
16. Opiola, K., & Ray, D. C. (2018). Child-centred play therapy with children who are dying. In L. C. Rubin (Ed.), *Handbook of medical play therapy and child life, interventions in clinical and medical settings.* Routledge.
17. Shaefer, C. E., & Drewes, A. A. (2013). *The therapeutic powers of play: 20 core agents of change.* John Wiley & Sons.
18. Jennings, S. (1999). *Introduction to developmental play therapy.* Jessica Kingsley.
19. Renshaw, K., Parson, J. & Zimmer, T. (2019). *Holistic play development.* Graphic, Deakin University.

20. Dempsey, S. (2008). *Extreme parenting: Parenting your child with a chronic illness. [adobe digital editions]*. Jessica Kingsley Publishers.
21. Niethammer, D. (2012). *Speaking honestly with sick and dying children and adolescents: Unlocking the silence*. The Johns Hopkins University Press.
22. Bluebond-Langner, M. (1978). *The private worlds of dying children*. Princeton University Press.
23. Doka, K. J. (1996). The cruel paradox: Children who are living with life threatening illnesses. In C. A. Corr & D. M. Corr (Eds.), *Handbook of childhood death and bereavement. [adobe digital editions]*. Springer Publishing Company.
24. Hubbuck, C. (2009). *Play for sick children: Play specialists in hospitals and beyond*. Jessica Kingsley Publishers.
25. Rae, W. A., & Sullivan, J. R. (2005). A review of play interventions for hospitalised children. In L. A. Reddy, T. M. Files-Hall, & C. E. Schaefer (Eds.), *Empirically based play therapy interventions for children*. American Psychological Association.
26. Harbeck-Weber, C., & McKee, D. H. (1995). Prevention of emotional and behavioural distress in children experiencing hospitalisation and chronic illness. In M. C. Roberts (Ed.), *Handbook of paediatric psychology* (2nd ed.). Guilford Press.
27. Hilliard, R. E. (2005). Music therapy in hospice and palliative care: A review of the empirical data. *Evidence-Based Contemporary and Alternative Medicine, 2*(2), 173–178.
28. Hartley, N. (2014). End of life care: A guide for therapists, artists and art therapists. *Jessica Kingsley Publishers*.
29. Brewster, A. B. (1982). Chronically ill hospitalised Children's concepts of their illness. *American Academy of Paediatrics, 69*(3), 355–362.
30. Tew, K. (2010). Filial therapy with parents of chronically ill children. In J. N. Baggerly, D. C. Ray, & S. C. Bratton (Eds.), *Child-centred play therapy research* (pp. 295–309). John Wiley & Sons.
31. Bluebond-Langner, M. (1996). *In the shadow of illness: Parents and siblings of the chronically ill child*. Princeton University Press.
32. Lane, C. (2013). Meeting the needs of siblings of children with life-limiting illness. *Art and Science, 26*(3), 16–20.
33. Meyer, D., & Vadasy, P. (2008). *Sibshops: Workshops for siblings of children with special needs*. Brookes Publishing.
34. Glazer-Waldman, H. G., Zimmerman, J., Landreth, G., & Norton, D. (1996). Filial therapy with parents of chronically ill children. In G. L. Landreth, L. E. Homeyer, G. Glover, & D. S. Sweeney (Eds.), *Play therapy interventions with children's problems* (pp. 65–68). Jason Aronson Inc.

Conclusion

Natalie A. Hadiprodjo, Judi A. Parson, and Belinda J. Dean

Children in the health care system may present with a range of physical, psychosocial and emotional needs. Health care experiences can be stressful for both children and their caregivers. Illness or injury may result in significant changes to a child's life including a change in daily routines, separation from family members and friends, changes in capabilities, and the need to adjust to new and strange people, places and experiences. The child may also endure uncomfortable or painful medical procedures. Whilst the immediate physical needs may be viewed as the most pressing in a health or medical context, easing a child's psychological distress is also vital to a child's overall health and wellbeing and in guarding against medical trauma.

This text has been written with the health care professional in mind, with a view to supporting developmentally sensitive nursing and allied health care by integrating the therapeutic powers of play into child and adolescent health care provision. Play is understood as a child's way of communicating and therefore it makes sense to integrate play into nursing and allied health care as a developmentally appropriate means of communicating with children. Children naturally use play to process and make sense of their world and experiences. If an adult intends to connect and communicate with a child, they must be willing to engage with the child via their preferred means of communication. Health care professionals involved in a child's care may utilise playful approaches to support children and families and ease the fear and anxiety children may experience in relation to medical procedures and/or hospital admissions.

N. A. Hadiprodjo (✉) · J. A. Parson · B. J. Dean
School of Health and Social Development, Deakin University, Geelong, VIC, Australia
e-mail: natalie.hadiprodjo@deakin.edu.au

J. A. Parson et al. (eds.), *Integrating Therapeutic Play Into Nursing and Allied Health Practice*, https://doi.org/10.1007/978-3-031-16938-0_16

Play can be utilised therapeutically as a tool to facilitate communication, support emotional wellness, enhance social relationships and increase personal strengths. Play can assist in reducing anxiety, eliciting positive emotions and building resilience and coping. Play can also be used to support positive relationships between caregivers and children, and the health care professional and the child. An understanding of attachment theory may also assist the health care professional in tailoring treatment to the child and responding with compassion to stressed caregivers and children within the health care setting. It is important that health care professionals also take time to reflect on their own attachment experiences, their motivations for working within paediatric health care, and their own attitude towards and experience of play.

Understanding a child's stage of development can help the health care professional consider the type of therapeutic play appropriate for a child. Like other facets of development, play is recognised as a sequentially developing ability that can be aligned with the child's age and stage of life. From the perspective of Erikson's stages of psychosocial development, play may also assist children in successfully navigating the crisis that comes with each stage of development, leading to the virtues of hope, will, purpose, competence and fidelity. Play-based approaches can be placed on a continuum from fully child-led or non-directive to adult-facilitated educative play. Play-based strategies may vary across this continuum from encouraging and creating opportunities for normative free play within the health care setting, to utilising play to help children prepare for hospitalisation, or developing play-based distraction techniques for use during medical procedures. For children who have experienced medical trauma or who are struggling with the emotional facets of illness or injury, play-based therapies such as Play Therapy or Filial Therapy may be beneficial.

A compassionate health care professional must also have the capacity to walk in the shoes of the child and see the world through their eyes. A health care practitioner who acknowledges the importance of play for the child and who is willing to engage in play-based approaches in the health care setting may prove a valuable companion for the Jesse's and Evan's of the world as they traverse their medical journeys through the challenges of allergy assessment and Botox injections. A health care professional who takes time to listen to a child's play may find this provides a unique glimpse into the child's world and how they perceive their medical condition and care. Furthermore, health care professionals who engage with children in an age-appropriate manner and 'speak' with children through their natural language of play, may enhance coping, resiliency and healing in children.

Printed in the United States
by Baker & Taylor Publisher Services